LABOR

SHARED EXPERIENCES
from the
DELIVERY ROOM

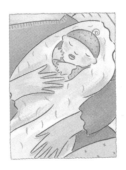

Edited by Ann-Marie Giglio

WORKMAN PUBLISHING • NEW YORK

For
my mother
and my daughters

The stories collected here represent a sampling of possible childbirth experiences
and are not intended as medical advice. Read them for inspiration,
for entertainment, for enlightenment, but not for instructions.

Library of Congress Cataloging-in-Publication Data
Labor day: tales from the delivery room:
32 personal accounts of labor and delivery/edited by Ann-Marie Giglio.
p.   cm.
ISBN 0-7611-0242-6
1. Labor (Obstetrics)—Anecdotes. 2. Childbirth—Anecdotes
I. Giglio, Ann-Marie.
RG652.L325 1999
618.4—DC21   99-18412
                                                      CIP

WORKMAN PUBLISHING COMPANY, INC.
708 Broadway
New York, NY 10003-9555

First printing July 1999
10 9 8 7 6 5 4 3 2 1

Acknowledgments

This book would not have been possible without the incredible generosity, enthusiasm, and support of its contributors. Even the people who responded to my queries but never sent a story made an important contribution to the book because their interest and feedback always buoyed me, often when I needed it most.

Without complaint, people worked with me through the sometimes lengthy process of editing their stories. They gave freely the intimate details of their experience, and they willingly struggled to find words for the indescribable, all for the good of the manuscript, because they shared my belief in the need for this book. It is unfortunate that every story we worked on did not fit into the final draft. Thank you, each of you, for helping me to create this anthology. I hope you are pleased with the result of our efforts.

I must also thank the people who posted my queries in their offices or publications, also supporting this process.

Thank you, Peter Workman, for assembling such a refined and energetic staff.

And thank you, Mom, for reminding me to follow my passions and forget about the laundry.

Contents

Preface

As a woman approaches the end of her first pregnancy, her focus tends to shift to labor and delivery. She wonders what it will be like and if she will be able to handle it. And it's no wonder she's uncertain. All too often, the labors we hear about are the eye-popping horror stories. But the truth is that most births are perfectly normal. I said normal, not easy.

A friend of mine calls the most difficult part of birth "Labor Land": the stretch of time when your entire reality is composed of contractions—the one you just had, the one you're having now, and the one you're anticipating. It usually strikes just before the pushing stage, when you're almost—almost—completely dilated. This is slippery terrain, where women tend to lose it. We scream. We moan. Some of us say nothing at all. The amazing thing is that we return to tell the tale.

And it is a tale that needs telling. People tend to spotlight the baby, both before and after its birth. But birth itself is wondrous and amazing. Squeezing that infant out of that tiny hole is seemingly impossible. It is a grand accomplishment, requiring women to defy their own limits. How do we do it?

Unfortunately, it is rare to witness birth today. For most of us, the first birth we experience is that of our own first child. So we go into labor, that vast unknown, harboring varying degrees of trepidation.

The how-to books present a clinical description of what labor ought to be like: what I call laboratory labor. Average first-time length: 12 to 14 hours. Stages: three. Timing and counting: important. Yet we are never given any clear sense of what labor feels like, exactly, or how to know it has actually started. How do we define a true labor contraction? And what if our contractions are never precisely five minutes apart?

This book is a collection of real labor stories, told by the fathers and caregivers, as well as the mothers, in their own voices. The storytellers attempt to answer these questions and to describe the indescribable. They tell of physical exertion, anxiety, pain, difficult decisions, surprising responses, and ultimately, success and joy.

To find the storytellers, I wrote letters and sent posters to national magazines, university writing programs, professional journals, newsletters, and the offices of doctors and midwives. I searched the Internet for bulletin boards where I posted requests. I spoke to family, friends, neighbors, and strangers. I received responses from hundreds of people, and they all wanted passionately to tell their stories.

Their accounts remind us that giving birth is bloody, sweaty, hard work. Often, it takes a very long time. And it hurts. It hurts us and it hurts our partners who watch, unable to carry the burden for even one moment. The stories also show that labor may cause us to do things without warning, things we never imagined we would, often in front of strangers. We scream, curse, lose our inhibitions. Or we may become silent, focus our energy inward.

Many of the stories show that giving birth can be a transforming experience, one that reveals unknown strengths and teaches invaluable lessons. They also remind us that our expectations may have little or nothing to do with the outcome.

Afterward, some of us may be embarrassed or disappointed because it was not the birth we'd hoped for. The baby is born, but we're dripping sweat and blood, still having contractions. We're exhausted. We're grateful it's over. All we want to do is sleep. Pretty tears aren't trickling down our cheeks. We're not bonding immediately with our infant as we are expected to. Or we might be sobbing openly, shouting with joy, melting with love.

If these stories show us only one thing, it's that labor is truly individual. The goal is the same—dilation and delivery—but not the path. So no reader's birth experience will be exactly the same as any of the stories told in this book. Because the confluence of events that end a gestation occur in different order for different people, we cannot predict when labor will begin. Nor can we predict how long it will last or when it will end. But we can take comfort from the knowledge that there are so many different ways of responding to and experiencing childbirth, and that even the unexpected is "normal." As one storyteller writes, "Birth is like a marriage. You have to know what you want but be prepared for anything." For this reason, I have tried to include stories not ordinarily heard, as well as some familiar ones, in hopes that readers will find it useful to have read about a range of experiences before they begin their own labor.

However, none of these stories is a recipe. Nothing in this book should be read as a proven method or a prescription or even a suggestion as to what is right for you. In fact, what these stories show is that there is no one correct way to labor or to deliver a baby. Giving birth, not our method or our response, is what unites us. Some people would find a medically managed birth suffocating; others would suffer without it. We must trust ourselves to discover what works for us and for our baby.

I hope that collectively these stories resound as a symphony of possibilities and that you find strength and inspiration in them. These storytellers offer you their support. They are here to reassure you that yes, labor is difficult, but you can and will find your own way.

If you have already given birth, I hope these stories will help you reconnect with your experience and give you pause for reflection. Some of the storytellers in this collection found the act of telling their labor stories personally illuminating. One father's story magnified for him the moment when, after ten years together, he and his wife turned a corner in their marriage and went from being a couple to being parents. A mother's story reaffirmed for her the strong sense of accomplishment she had felt. Another mother was able to come to terms with her emergency first birth by writing about her beautiful second birth. For other mothers, telling their stories sparked a new recognition of how giving birth had empowered them. It gave them the chance to see exactly how they had taken that giant step from woman to mother.

Many of the people who shared their stories with me told me that whether or not I used the story in the book, they were pleased to have a record of it, and they thanked me for the opportunity to create one. I hope you, too, will be inspired to record the details of your story on the pages reserved for you at the book's end. Revel in your accomplishment. Take a fine, close look at it. For once you have given birth or witnessed birth, you are changed.

POEM TO EASE CHILDBIRTH

In the house with the tortoise chair
She will give birth to the pearl
To the beautiful feather.

In the house of the goddess who sits on a tortoise,
She will give birth to the necklace of pearls
To the beautiful feathers we are.

There she sits on the tortoise,
Swelling to give us birth.

On your way, On your way,
Child be on your way to me here,
You whom I made new.

Come here child . . . Come be pearl . . . be beautiful
feather.

—Anonymous, Aztec tribe

1

Now I Can Do Anything!

*Jennifer is a registered nurse now working in a newborn
intensive care unit in a Tulsa, Oklahoma hospital. Her
husband, Jon, age 32 is a student of elementary education.
Jennifer writes, "When I hear of other women's labors and
births, many say they were disappointed. But mine turned
out almost exactly the way I had hoped it would."
Despite her professional experience, though, Jennifer
almost didn't make it to the hospital on time!*

My first daughter, Susanna, was born in July 1993. I still think of her birth nearly every day. It was the happiest, most empowering day of my life. It went so fast, though, that I felt a bit cheated. I didn't get to use all the relaxation techniques and visualizations I'd been practicing.

I take some credit for Susanna's birth turning out so well, because I did everything I could to make that happen. I read everything by Sheila Kitzinger; *Natural Childbirth the Bradley Way;* and Adrienne Lieber-

3

man's *Easing Labor Pain*. I stretched and did yoga every day, and drank herbal tea the last six weeks. Most importantly, I carefully picked my caregiver. I wanted to be as informed as I could about choosing the person who had power over such an important event in my life.

Selecting the right caregiver is crucial in helping a woman get the birth experience she wants. I'm an RN; when I had Susanna I was working in a hospital nursery and obstetrics unit, so I was familiar with the styles of many doctors. Unfortunately, their patients rarely are. I'd see patients come in with elaborate, typewritten birth plans and feel sorry for them because I knew their doctors, and I knew the patients weren't going to get what they wanted. Birth plans so often become meaningless when the real chain of events begins. You need to find a caregiver for whom a written birth plan would be redundant, someone whose basic ideas about childbirth are compatible with yours.

When I first got pregnant, I'd heard of people who gave birth at home and I thought they were crazy and irresponsible. After all, I'd been at deliveries that had gone bad in a flash. But as I read more, I learned that sometimes deliveries go bad because of what happens in the hospital—the anesthesia, the inability to move around during labor, the lithotomy position (lying on the back with legs in stirrups). So I became interested in a home birth and called the American College of Nurse Midwives to get some names. They told me that in Oklahoma nurse midwives cannot attend home births. But they did give me the name of a board-certified male obstetrician who is also a certified midwife.

At my first appointment, I asked him many questions and felt very reassured: he didn't do routine episiotomies; he had a very low C-section rate; he wouldn't automatically rule out a vaginal delivery for a breech baby. Then he said that my husband Jon could deliver the baby if he wanted to, and offered to guide Jon through it. Wow! I'd never even considered that possibility. As it turned out, things happened too quickly for any of us to remember to get Jon some gloves, let alone deliver the baby.

When I was a couple of days past my due date, and had already lost my mucous plug a week earlier, of course, I was wondering when this baby was coming. That Monday morning I'd gotten up, determined to get something going. I started banging around the house, not so subtly trying to get Jon to wake up and join me in this endeavor. He did wake up and was not too happy about it; it was his day off, and he likes to sleep in.

YOU NEED A CAREGIVER WHOSE BASIC IDEAS ABOUT CHILDBIRTH ARE COMPATIBLE WITH YOURS.

We had a fight, which ended with my crying, "I'm never going to have this baby!" I also told him not to bother coming to my 3:00 doctor's appointment with me, but, since he's not the jerk I was trying to make him out to be, he came anyway.

The doctor examined me and, to my great delight, told me I was dilated to about 3 centimeters and was "stretchy; ready to go at any time." I was elated and not mad at Jon anymore. I kept repeating in wonder all evening, "I'm 3 centimeters!" We walked around the mall until my feet started hurting. We were hungry, so we decided to go home and fix a big special meal and watch a movie. In retrospect, what we should have done was get some rest. At the time we thought that even though I was 3 centimeters dilated, since I wasn't feeling any contractions, I could be at 3 for a long, long time. It was my first baby, after all.

So we bought shrimp, corn on the cob, salad greens, and garlic bread, and we rented a movie. After dinner we watched the movie. Throughout the evening I had started to feel some contractions, like menstrual cramps, nothing that seemed regular, and certainly nothing worth timing. During the movie, I suddenly felt one strong contraction that really caught my attention because it didn't feel anything like cramps; it actually felt as if something was being forced open, and I knew that something was my cervix! But there was just that one, so I didn't even mention it to Jon. When the movie was over, around 1:30 a.m., I went to the bathroom, came back to the living room, and then my water broke in a big gush.

That was the strangest moment for both of us, I think. Suddenly, labor became real. This was really going to happen. Jon went to get towels, while I went back to the bathroom to look at the fluid and make sure it wasn't stained with meconium. Meconium, a greenish-brown substance, is the baby's first bowel movement. In overdue babies, the risk of a first bowel movement in utero is greater. If a baby has swallowed meconium, or swallows some during a vaginal birth, I knew a serious infection could result. So, if I saw any sign of meconium, intervention would be warranted. Fortunately, the fluid was clear. I took a quick shower and we went to bed around 2:00. My plan was to get some sleep and then go get checked by the doctor again in the morning. But we'd only been in bed about 15 minutes when my contractions started, and it quickly became evident that I was not going to be able to rest.

The contractions did not build up slowly, as the books said they would. They were intense and furious immediately, and no more than five minutes apart. We never even formally timed them; they were just always there. I desperately wanted to find the heating pad; we tore the closet apart looking for it; but when I used it, the heat was too uncomfortable. Jon tried to rub my feet and back (which is what I had firmly told him I'd want, back in the innocence of our Bradley classes), but I couldn't remain still. I hung over the back of the sofa or knelt on the bed, doubling myself over the pillows trying to catch hold of each contraction to better manage it.

I think I did well. I remember a couple of times I started to hyperventilate and Jon breathed with me to slow me down, but I'm proud of the way I made it through labor. Even if I had thought it might help to yell or scream, I don't think I would have had the energy. All my energy was focused inside my body, on each coming tidal wave of pain. I didn't even worry about the baby; I just trusted that it wasn't in distress.

We should have gone to the hospital sooner. I was a nurse, I was well read, I should have known better. But even though I had a pretty good idea that things were progressing rapidly, the labor was so intense that I couldn't imagine getting in the car and having to sit still for the 15-minute ride. Jon wasn't aware of how fast it was going; he just knew that a first labor was supposed to last about 14 hours and was wondering how I would manage without an epidural for the next 11 hours or so. When I began shaking and couldn't hear anything Jon was saying, I knew I was in transition. That's when I got scared that we'd never get to the hospital in time, and I wondered whether we should call 911. Instead, I called the hospital, told them we were coming, and told Jon that we needed to go.

But first I insisted on taking a quick shower, because I now had some bloody show. I got on my hands and knees and let the water hit my back and it felt wonderful. I wished I'd remembered the shower trick earlier. I probably would have stayed in the shower forever, but Jon dragged me out and helped me into some clothes. (Bless his heart, he didn't know how to fit the sanitary pad into my panties; it seems obvious, but he stuck it on sideways.) Then he helped me into the car, which he'd backed all the way up to our front porch so I wouldn't have to walk any further than necessary.

I remember the ride to the hospital as being very bumpy, which is odd, because I know those streets are smooth. By this time, the contractions had decreased in intensity and were further apart, and I was feeling the need to push. I remembered to pant, which really did help keep me from pushing. Jon, still unaware of what was going on (I wasn't feeling very communicative), told me I was breathing too fast. I said, "You don't get it. If I don't pant, I'll push." That was when he realized how close we were to having our baby. He pulled into the emergency room entrance, went inside to find a wheelchair for me, pushed me to the clerk, then went back outside to park the car.

An ER nurse took me to Labor and Delivery, where Judy, one of my favorite nurses, was waiting. She quickly got me into bed and checked me. I recall her surprised words: "The head is right there . . . Jennifer, let's have a baby!" She called out to another nurse to call my doctor. Jon was coming down the hall at that time and heard her saying: ". . . and tell him to move his butt!" Now Jon *really* knew what was happening! He walked in, took a look between my legs (I was now quite happy to be lying in bed) and saw the top of the baby's blond head just waiting to be pushed out.

Judy said the doctor was about 20 minutes away. I panted and breathed and managed to hold off until he arrived. He walked in, took a look, said, "The position's perfect," put on a pair of gloves, and told me to push. (I had actually already pushed a few times, involuntarily. It was incredible. My body was doing the pushing; I had nothing to do with it. I know some people say they never felt the urge to push. For me, there was no way I could have stopped it.)

The most pain I ever felt was when the head crowned, but I knew it wouldn't last long. When the head was out, Jon looked at me and said, "It's beautiful!" I'll never forget his face; he looked so happy and so excited. Then he and Judy held my legs up as I pushed the rest of the baby out; I can still remember that slippery, slithery feeling between my thighs. Judy said, "It's a girl!" which is what we'd both been hoping for. It was 5:37 a.m., Tuesday.

A few minutes later, I delivered the placenta, which we took home to plant in our garden. Susanna nursed eagerly right away, but I still bled a lot immediately afterward, so Judy gave me a shot of methergine and then started an IV to give me some Pitocin, to help shrink my uterus. I hadn't torn at all, and I was up and walking around right away. I felt great! We left the hospital that afternoon.

Later that day, our families came to our house to see the baby, and we ordered pizza. When they left, the three of us crashed.

Susanna's birth turned out almost exactly as I had hoped: no hanging around the hospital when I wasn't in active labor, no drugs, no episiotomy, no lengthy hospital stay, no problems for either one of us. Looking back, though, it's kind of scary to think of how many things could have gone wrong. I am extremely thankful and grateful that we had such a wonderful experience.

Since then, it sometimes seems that I can literally feel, tingling in my cells, the power of being female, passed down to me through centuries and centuries of DNA. I now feel a personal connection to the women on my family's genealogical charts that I never felt before. Before, they were just interesting names, but now they are real people to me. They must have experienced the same birth and mothering feelings I have. It makes me wish I could talk to them.

Birth was also empowering for me. After Susanna was born, I read an article in *Shape* magazine about a woman dogsledder. The article said the woman had "killed a grizzly, raced in minus 62 degrees, and given birth without painkillers." I was first startled, and then pleased, that someone had ranked natural childbirth on the same level as killing a grizzly bear. That really made me feel strong and powerful. I, who was always the wimp in gym class whom nobody wanted on their team, felt vindicated.

Now I believe I can do anything.

Waiting for Godot

*Rini was a 28-year-old graduate student studying sociology
and her husband, Larry, 31, was a graphic design student
when they had their first child in a hospital in Chicago. Rini had
her heart set on a natural birth. However, one week after
her due date, when she failed the non-stress test and the bio-physical
profile, labor was induced. Nonetheless she writes:
"Nutshell: Healthy baby. Happy new family is born."*

W hen I was about 37 weeks pregnant, I started to get excited, thinking about how it could be "any day now." (I don't know why I let myself do this; I *know* that many first-time mothers deliver late, but I couldn't help myself.) Of course, a person can maintain that level of excitement only for so long.

After the actual due date came and went, I sort of gave up on the idea of ever going into labor. I decided to just get on with my life, big belly or not. So I didn't hesitate to schedule my dissertation proposal hearing for five days after the baby's due date. I figured *something* was going to happen that week: either I'd have a baby or defend my proposal (or maybe both).

11

My July 20 proposal hearing went very well, but I had no signs of going into labor. At least I got one thing accomplished. The next day, Friday, I was told to "drop into" the hospital for a non-stress test (NST) early in the morning, and then I had planned to do a bunch of errands. I wasn't going to let impending labor stop me. Well, there was no "dropping in" for the NST. I had to wait for more than an hour in a very disorganized place before I was finally seated in a tiny room for the test (unfortunately, Larry had to wait outside). Finally, a nurse came in and placed a stretchy belt around my tummy and positioned a transducer where we could hear "Baby Godot's" heartbeat loud and clear. (For me, pregnancy was about waiting and hoping and wondering if the baby would ever come. Since that's about all I got out of the Beckett play, *Waiting for Godot*, "Baby Godot" became our in utero nickname for our baby.)

The test routinely takes half an hour, but it can be shorter if the baby moves around a lot right away. But after 20 minutes on the machine, the only movement Godot had made was to hiccup, and apparently that doesn't count. The technician seemed a little concerned, but with only a few minutes left on the clock, Godot made the requisite three movements within the 30-minute time period. Finally, it was over.

I stopped in at the midwives' office to show them the results. Pat noted the baby's three kicks at the end and was enthusiastic, but because of the long quiet spell, she wanted to show the strip to the doctor. She ran out to meet the doctor and came back in a few minutes to tell us that he wanted me to have a bio-physical profile (BPP), a more thorough fetal monitoring test. It was beginning to look like I might have trouble getting all my errands done.

We had time to run out for lunch before the test, so we did, in the hopes that some fuel might help Godot make a more impressive showing. While we ate, Godot kicked a lot, and I wasn't worried. (He had kicked both before and after the NST, so I figured he was just caught napping.)

When we returned for the BPP, again we had to wait a really long time. Finally, we were shown to a small dark room. The ultrasound was fun at first—we could see Godot's fingers and toes and ribs. We didn't know the sex of the baby and the technician peeked around a bit for us. She said she didn't see anything, so it was probably a girl. But . . . perhaps those were testicles? Maybe a boy? Hard to say.

Pretty soon the ultrasound got to be less fun. Godot wasn't moving again. That didn't bother me so much, but it bothered the technician. She started making me nervous. She kept jiggling my tummy and encouraging the baby to do something, then fretting when he didn't move. This went on for half an hour. Finally she left the room with a grave expression on her face and didn't return for a long time.

After a while, I was told to get dressed, and then was called to the phone to talk to the midwives. My midwife, Charity, said frankly, "It's time to have this baby." Wow, did I freak out. She said the baby was "looking old," he had only scored a 4 out of 8 on the BPP, and that I should just walk straight over to Labor and Delivery for an induction. Larry was watching me as I listened to Charity, but he didn't know what she was saying and when he saw me break down in tears, he felt his heart skip a beat.

Why was I crying? Partly from shock and fear for the baby, and partly from disappointment that this wasn't going to be the labor I had

13

wanted. But it was also largely from joy. I was finally going to have a baby. I had sort of emotionally written off the possibility of having a baby, so despite all evidence to the contrary, this was like a big surprise to me.

After taking a few minutes to cry some more, we went to Labor and Delivery. This was not how I planned on arriving! Instead of carrying a suitcase packed with my nightie and slippers, I was holding a bunch of articles for photocopying, and my professor's comments on my dissertation proposal!

After I had checked into my room, they attached an external monitor and the baby looked terrific. In fact, the baby looked so good that the staff started wondering why I was there. So they called the on-call doctor to redo the BPP, to see if maybe we could wait after all. This time, Godot did much better from the start. The only concern this doctor had during the exam was that the amniotic fluid seemed low. However, she had to leave for an emergency a few minutes into the exam and well before she could find all eight points for my baby. Since it was already five days past my due date, the low level of amniotic fluid was enough to raise a red flag. So they remained set on induction.

When the doctor returned, she gave me an internal exam and while doing it, she announced, "If you feel pain, it's because I'm stripping your membranes." At the time this made me angry. I considered that to be a medical procedure, and I felt I should have been asked for consent. Looking back, though, I'm sure that with a little thought, I would have given my consent. I was already on the road to an induced labor and this was a low-intervention way to get things started. And get things started it did. I started contracting right away, with contractions less than five minutes apart. However, they didn't last. Gradually they slowed down and finally stopped.

Dinner and a long walk with Larry did not seem to help. So Charity announced that it was time for "vitamin P"—Pitocin. At about 8:00 p.m., I was hooked up to the IV and the external monitor, given a Pitocin drip, and my contractions started again.

At 9:00, Larry and I noticed that the baby's heart rate was slowing a bit during each contraction, down to maybe 100. We asked the nurse about it and she said that was normal. However, five minutes later, the heart rate dropped to 80 during a contraction and the nurse came bolting down the hall with my midwife—apparently this was *not* normal. They shut off the Pitocin and told me to roll right and left, and sit up and lie down. Finally, the heart-rate decelerations stopped. At around 10:00, I was still only 2 centimeters dilated, so Charity wanted to have my waters broken so that an internal monitor could be installed, as well as a catheter to replenish my amniotic fluid. Having my waters broken hurt like hell, since I was hardly dilated at all.

By 11:00 p.m., I was having regular contractions about 30 seconds long and three minutes apart. By midnight, I was starting to vocalize my discomfort. Labor was no fun; between the contractions I was in full-body trembling, which is no way to rest. It was a killer. Finally, at 5:00 a.m. I had to give up on the Bradley method. This was not the natural labor I had planned for at all. Because of the IV and the internal monitor, I hadn't been out of bed the whole time. No walking, no showers, no getting on all-fours for me. I was at 5 centimeters and had been for a long time. I asked Charity for an epidural and, frankly, she looked relieved and supported my decision entirely.

At 5:30 a.m. the anesthesiologist arrived. Though I had been anti-epidural, I referred to him as "my hero" when he entered the room. Getting the epidural in was no problem. There was pain when the needle went in, but it was such a different kind of pain from the contractions, I appreciated the variety. I was now fully wired. Connected to me, I had the Pitocin drip, the epidural, amniotic replenishment fluid, a glucose drip, an internal monitor, an oxygen mask, a blood pressure cuff, and, of course, the TV remote control.

BEFORE I WENT INTO LABOR, I HAD MY HEART DEAD SET AGAINST USING AN EPIDURAL, BUT NOW I THANK GOD I HAD THE OPTION AVAILABLE TO ME.

Before I went into labor, I had my heart dead set against using an epidural, but now I thank God I had the option available to me. It changed everything and it turned out to be one of the few positive aspects of my whole labor experience. For the past eight hours, the only thing I had said was "Oooowwww!" Suddenly, I was the life of the party. I was cracking jokes and talking up a storm. The full-body trembling went away entirely, and I was able to fall asleep. An hour earlier, no one would have believed that I would be able to sleep! I don't know how I would have survived without it—not as cheerfully, that's for sure.

The midwives changed shifts in the morning. When Joan came in to replace Charity at around 8:30 on Saturday, July 22, she decided to do an internal exam to see how I was doing. She surprised us all by looking up and saying, "We're having a baby." Once again, I started crying. (I swear, it was always surprising to learn I was having a baby up until . . . well, it still is!) Joan told Charity that she deserved to catch the baby, so they both hung around for the birth, which I thought was really neat.

Now, because we were a week postdate and, even more, because of the low level of amniotic fluid—the midwives gave us a serious lecture. They were pretty sure there was meconium in the fluid and that it was thick. They told us that in this event, the baby would be rushed off by the pediatricians for suctioning and would not be delivered onto my stomach. Might as well burn our birth plan now.

After all the proper personnel—two midwives, the anesthesiologist, an RN, and a team from the neonatal unit, ready to deal with meconium aspiration if necessary—were assembled, Joan and Charity told me to start pushing. I told them they were nuts. I had no urge to push and no idea how to do it. Joan replied sternly that I had been practicing all my life—it was just like having a bowel movement. (My sweet, perky midwives suddenly turned into no-nonsense, bossy drill sergeants when it came time to push.) I snapped back that I didn't even know where my butt was, let alone how to push anything out of it. (The epidural was still very much in effect, and I was numb down there.) However, I closed my eyes and bore down. I couldn't feel my legs, but each midwife took hold of one and pushed them, knees bent, back toward my chest. Right away they started yelling that they could see the head. I could hear Larry, too, in a very strange tone of voice, saying something like, "Ohmigod, it's right there! Wow! It's coming!" This was *extremely* encouraging, so determination set in and I pushed like crazy. I never did open my eyes. I didn't want any distractions. At one point, they asked me if I wanted to feel the head or see it in a mirror but my feeling was "Not a chance! I'm busy, people! Just leave me to get this task done, please."

So I was pushing but not feeling. I didn't feel the burn of crowning or the slimy sploosh of the rest of the body, but within half an hour of starting to push, they all shouted, "It's clear!" referring to the amniotic fluid and then they put this little purple thing on my stomach at 10:22 a.m. Finally, I opened my eyes. And there was my baby! Larry was leaning over me, all teary-eyed. I just kept saying, "Oh my god, a baby! My baby!" Somebody shouted out that it was a boy, but that little "surprise" of delivery really didn't compare at all to the surprise I felt at actually having a baby. He was so little and . . . well, there he was, this *person*, who hadn't been there a moment before.

So, after all the anxiety, Jasper scored 9 and 9 on his Apgars. He weighed in at 6 pounds, 13 ounces, which is small for my family (my sister's baby was almost 11 pounds!), but he's been packing in the breast milk since then and is catching up to us upper-percentile types pretty quickly.

And that's the end of the beginning. Really, the most wonderful part of the story is everything that follows.

There's No Place Like Home

*Valeri was a 21-year-old secretary, and her husband
Robert a 20-year-old electrician, when they had their
first child at home, in Benicia, California. They went on to
birth three more children at home. Valeri is now a writer.*

My due date had come and gone, and I was getting huge. I felt massive, thudding through my house. It felt as if I would be pregnant forever. As soon as I would become so thoroughly discouraged as to contemplate begging for an induction, a round of contractions would strike: 20 minutes, 15 minutes, 10 minutes apart. Each time, I was certain this was it. But then the contractions would peter out, only to begin again in a day or so, starting another cycle of false hope.

I awoke in a wonderful mood on March 30. I felt strong and positive. It was five days past my due date. "Maybe today," I thought. My midwife, Hsui-li (*Sho-lee*) called to check on me. Since I was having a few contractions, she said I could try taking some castor oil. I knew to

19

expect a laxative effect, but not to what extent. Hsui-li did advise me to drink it with plenty of fluids.

Happily, I waddled off to the drugstore just blocks from my house for the magical potion. It was a beautiful spring morning, very warm, the sun shining, the blossoms sweet on the trees. I tried to make mental notes of it all; in case this was to be the big day, I wanted to remember everything. The clerk at the store smiled knowingly at me as I paid for my purchase, but neither of us said a word.

I couldn't get home fast enough. I took a dose of the awful stuff in a glass of orange juice. It tasted wretched, a taste I can still recall. I drank it and then waited, pacing. Within 45 minutes, terrible cramps and diarrhea started, along with light sporadic contractions. The tremendous pressure and activity in my lower belly made it difficult to separate the various sensations. The contractions were nothing like menstrual cramps. They were stronger, deeper, knottier feelings. They were mildly painful, and perfect, miniature replications of the stronger contractions that would come later. But I didn't have much faith in them. I had been fooled before.

I called my doula, Barbara, to tell her what I had done. She suggested that if things didn't really get moving soon, I might want to take another dose of the castor oil. I waited another hour and when labor hadn't progressed as I had hoped, I took more, this time mixing it with a protein shake. The effect was immediate. I began having contractions every 12 minutes, lasting 45 seconds and gaining in intensity. I had done it! I was full of anticipation. My baby would be born soon. It was 2:00 in the afternoon and I didn't have any idea what awaited me. So far the contractions were completely tolerable, though mildly uncomfortable. I was determined to be the bravest new mother in the world.

I called my husband, Robert, at work to let him know my labor had started, but said not to rush home as I didn't need him yet. I promised I would call him if things got too hard for me to handle alone. I began preparing the house, changing sheets, gathering supplies for the birth, and doing last-minute cleaning. I took a wonderful, long shower with perfumed soap. I felt so alive. Everything was so vivid, every sight, every smell, each sensation was magnified tenfold. I didn't want to get out and stayed in the shower until the water grew cold.

The contractions were getting stronger and had become regular, each lasting about 60 seconds, with the interval closing by a few minutes each hour. Sometimes the interval was longer, which was a relief, but it also made me nervous that my labor might stop. The contractions began deep within my pelvis, just behind my pubic bone, and spread up and around my big belly, tightening. It felt the way muscles do after you've been working out too hard, as if the muscles were so taut they could explode. Hot and tight: that was my sense of a contraction.

I wanted to be pretty for the birth of our baby, so I put on makeup and curled my hair. It was getting increasingly difficult to ignore the contractions. By now I would have to stop whatever I was doing to follow the sensation through.

At about 6:00 p.m., I felt warm water running gently down my leg. My water had broken. A moment of reckoning. Now I knew this was really going to be it. Robert arrived home and I was so glad to see him. I had begun to feel a bit nervous about being alone. My neighbor came

21

by to check on me. He was so excited to discover my labor had started. He and Robert were staring at me and I found them too distracting after having spent the day alone, so I politely asked my neighbor to leave. I knew it was time to call my mother and Barbara. I was ready for their guidance and company.

The contractions were becoming painful, more intense, longer, deeper, stronger, hotter, and were requiring my full attention. I was certain that I must be dilated at least 5 centimeters, perhaps even more judging by the feel of the five-minute contractions I'd had for the last hour. When Barbara arrived at 7:00 and examined me, I was discouraged to find I was only 3½ centimeters dilated.

In the meantime, my mom had also arrived. I tried to stay as nonchalant as I could, chatting with her, talking on the phone, tackling the steep flight of stairs in our house. Climbing the stairs was actually therapeutic at that point. I felt less discomfort if I moved my body, and I felt more in control. I was no longer able to speak during the contractions, but I could move. I moved from place to place, all around the house, wandering, sort of pacing, stopping to sit now and then, then standing up again. It helped rid me of some nervous energy, I think.

The contractions were now coming every two minutes. I tried to relax in a warm bath, but the water didn't fully cover my belly and I felt claustrophobic in the tub. I sat through only two contractions before I got out.

Barbara continued to check my dilation and to monitor my vital signs. It was becoming hard to think straight. I was hot and sweaty even though everyone else was chilly. I was only wearing Robert's oversized shirt and a pair of socks, but at this point, I was burning up inside. The contractions seemed to give off heat, starting off nice and warm in my pelvis, spreading up my body, until finally my face was ablaze.

I began feeling nauseous and dizzy. When I was 5 centimeters dilated, I began to vomit after every couple of contractions. Each time, I felt momentarily relieved, though the relief didn't last long. It felt unfair that I should be sick when I was so busy dealing with the contractions. I camped out in the bathroom, on the cool tile. When I wasn't vomiting, I would sit on the toilet. I was comfortable sitting behind the closed door in privacy. Barbara would check on me, and sometimes rub my back or talk me through contractions. She assured me that the combination of toilet sitting and vomiting was helping me dilate faster.

I was moving along nicely, about a centimeter an hour. My mother and Robert sat quietly, waiting. Robert and I really didn't know what to expect. We had taken childbirth classes, but until you have actually gone through labor, there is nothing that can fully prepare you for it. I was so thankful to have Barbara there to help guide and reassure us.

At 10:40 p.m., three hours before the birth, when I was about 6 or 7 centimeters dilated I felt a new intensity to the sensations. The contractions now felt like a tight, thick rubber band around my middle, constricting tighter and tighter and then gradually loosening. I had been using a breathing pattern I'd devised to cope with the contractions, but that was no longer effective. I began thinking of them as tidal waves. First came the swell, gaining momentum and strength, sweeping me up in its powerful current, pulling me along. I was powerless to fight it; I had to surrender. Then, at the peak of each contraction, the wave would crash on the shore and slowly spread across the beach as the contraction dwindled away. I found that the less I fought the feeling, the less it hurt. The calmer I remained, the faster and easier the contractions seemed to pass. So I set my mind on being perfectly still and open to the sensations.

I soon began to visualize the contractions. I saw myself on a big, bright yellow surfboard, riding the waves out in the ocean. I've never surfed! Isn't that funny? But this vision helped me through several strong contractions. Visualizing became a very important coping tool.

THE THOUGHT OF HAVING AN ACTUAL BABY AT THE END OF ALL THIS SEEMED RIDICULOUS. EVERYTHING FELT SO BIZARRE AND SURREAL.

The second thing that helped tremendously was focusing entirely upon what was physically happening during a contraction. I imagined my uterus tightening and my cervix opening, allowing my baby to slide through. This helped me deal with the powerful feelings I was having, and prevented me from thinking it was all in vain. It reminded me what I was working for—a baby—which was surprisingly easy to forget. The thought of having an actual baby at the end of all this seemed ridiculous. Everything felt so bizarre and surreal.

During this time, I thought of all the other women who were also having babies, my sisters in birthing. Next, I wondered who was dying, but this was a fleeting thought, because I really didn't care. Suddenly, it came to me that I was all alone in this experience and I felt alone in the world. Even those in the room who loved me were separate from me and could not reach me. No one else could feel what I was feeling. No one else could get into the world I was in, and as much as I wished to, I certainly could not get out. I wondered if I might go insane. Had that ever happened?

Between contractions, I began to silently talk to myself, in full conversations. I had no sense of time. The contractions were running into one another. I felt very spacey. Robert, my mother, and Barbara all slipped in and out of my consciousness, their voices and faces like a dream. I could hear the sound of rain tapping on the window. When had it begun raining? Was I imagining it? No, it really was raining. Then, I heard them talking about how I was sleeping in between contractions, but I wasn't. I simply could not speak. I was paralyzed, too heavy and tired to respond, to even open my eyes. A contraction would come and drag me from wherever I was sitting, the rocking chair or the toilet, and I would walk. By now, we were all upstairs.

At nearly midnight, Hsui-li arrived. I had completely forgotten about her and didn't even know she had been called. We were all gathered in my bedroom, and when she walked in, I felt a bit of my composure fall away. I wanted to fall apart. Again, I wondered how the baby would get out if I lost my mind. I knew though, that the baby was coming, labor would continue, and that nature made no exception for the insanity plea.

I had been 7 centimeters when last checked and now I expected to be 8, but when Hsui-li checked me I was only 5. I wanted to scream. How could that be? How could I be going backward? I had been doing everything I was supposed to: moving around, relaxing, having faith in my body. Had Barbara's estimations been wrong? How could I possibly continue if I was only at 5 centimeters? Hsui-li said the baby was now in posterior position (facing my front instead of my back). I knew that posterior babies were harder to push out and sometimes had longer, more difficult labors. I wanted to cry. I wanted the whole thing stopped. Then, I remembered all the people who had told me I was crazy to have my baby at home. This inspired me to prove to them that I could do it. Also, I wanted to be brave for Robert and my mom, both of whom were somewhat nervous.

Barbara suggested I get on all fours to help the baby turn. I had been in labor 12 hours now, and I was very tired, so I just knelt on the floor and laid my arms and upper body across my bed. Oh, how I wanted a nap. I wanted labor to stop for just one hour so I could sleep. The two minutes between contractions were not enough rest and I felt so weak. All my energy was stolen by the pain.

By this point, I wanted everyone near me. I needed them, needed their energy. I would announce the onset of each contraction, believing that their knowledge of the contraction would somehow take the edge off of the pain. Hsui-li did acupressure, holding pressure points on my head quite firmly. I imagined the pain going out through my head into her hands, which helped. She reminded me to relax and I tried to melt into the floor.

When she checked me again, my water began to trickle some more. She began turning the baby internally, with one hand inside me and one on my belly. I kept saying that it hurt, hoping she would stop, but she kept on. A contraction came and I screamed or moaned to myself. I became lost in this sound, as if the sound and the pain were one and I existed within them. But when she finished, only seconds later, the baby was turned and I was completely dilated. She told me I could push now, whenever I felt like it.

I didn't have a physical urge to push, but was anxious to try. This was the moment I had been waiting for, to have some real control. I tried to get comfortable on the waterbed, which was difficult since it was sloshing around. My back was propped up with pillows, and Robert was at my side, holding my hand. At first I gave a tentative push. I could tell that wasn't going to get me anywhere, so I pushed again, with all my might, and felt my bottom half open up. I felt the baby begin to move through my pelvis, a slow rumble.

I began pushing at about 1:15 a.m. There was some commotion as last-minute supplies were being gathered, but I paid no attention to that. I was absorbed by my task. Once I had begun pushing, the contractions no longer hurt. Hsui-li knelt on the floor and Barbara sat on the edge of the bed, both facing me, while I was facing the side of the bed. I propped my legs up on Barbara and Hsui-li's hips on each side of me. My mother was taking pictures. I felt my body opening up wider and wider as the baby moved down, felt the burning, stinging, stretching of my perineum as the baby's head pushed from within. Robert was pouring olive oil on my perineum and it felt soothing and cool on the stretching skin. With each contraction, I pushed harder than with the one before. Barbara was feeding me ice chips. I became dependent upon these chips and would urgently call, "Ice, ice, ice!" between each push.

It wasn't that I even wanted the ice; it simply helped take my mind off the overwhelming burning sensation.

I could feel my pelvis separate as the baby moved down even further. Then she crowned! Barbara told me to touch my baby's head. I reached down and touched the warm, wrinkly, wet scalp. It didn't feel like a head at all. I didn't know what it felt like, I only knew I wanted it out. I began to laugh and cry simultaneously, overwhelmed with emotion, feelings I had never known before and will never forget, feelings that belong only to that night, only to birth. For a moment, it all made perfect sense, labor and birth and life. Within all the turmoil and buzzing of energy, there was an absolute peace. There was no time, there was no pain, all of life was suspended, held in that instant.

> **I BEGAN TO LAUGH AND CRY SIMULTANEOUSLY, OVERWHELMED WITH EMOTION, FEELINGS THAT BELONG ONLY TO THAT NIGHT, ONLY TO BIRTH. FOR A MOMENT, IT ALL MADE PERFECT SENSE, LABOR AND BIRTH AND LIFE.**

I panted so I wouldn't push too hard and tear my perineum. Hsui-li was helping ease the head out. Once it was out, I expected the body to just slip out. Instead, it was sliding out very slowly. I looked over my belly to see the baby. Hsui-li was unwinding this beautiful blue cord from the baby's neck. My baby was born. I lifted my shirt and a limp, little baby was placed on my belly. They began suctioning her until there were faint, gurgly cries. I let out a sigh. I asked if it was a boy or girl, but no one answered. They were too busy to check. It seemed like a long time before Hsui-li finally answered, "A girl." A daughter. Our daughter! "What will you name her?" she asked. "Brittany," I said. "Brittany Michelle." Robert kissed me. The next few moments were a blur of hugs and kisses and exclamations.

Then Robert cut the cord. I had been waiting for him to do it, watching. I always thought it very symbolic for the father to do this. I remember watching him prepare to make the cut, but I do not remember the actual cut, as if my mind blocked out the fact that the baby was now separate from me. She was now her own person.

As my mother swaddled little Brittany, the midwife coaxed the placenta out. I was tired and no longer wanted to push. After being convinced it wouldn't hurt, I gave one more big push and out it came. Then, the midwife helped clean me up, changed the sheets, and at last, handed me my baby to nurse. I was very awkward, not sure of what or how to do it, but the baby didn't seem to mind. She wasn't so sure herself.

We all just stared at her, so pure and perfect, marveling at her tiny little fingers, her perfect miniature features. She seemed the most beautiful baby ever born. She was gorgeous. How could we have created such a miracle? It was difficult to believe she had come from my body. It was on a prayer of thanks that we drifted off to sleep, me and my new family.

As the Pain Fades, the Miracle Fills In

Jen was 30 and her husband, Daniel, 33 at the time of their daughter's birth in a hospital in San Diego, California. She is an aerobics instructor and personal trainer, and he is an attorney.

Miriam was born December 29, 1994, on her daddy's birthday. My midwife had been telling me for months that the best way to induce labor was to have sex. I kept laughing it off. But, I didn't want to be late, and we did think that a last-minute tax deduction for the year would be nice. So when my husband Daniel came home from work on Wednesday evening and said that so and so from work had also told him that sex really would induce labor, we decided what the heck, let's try it.

The minute we finished making love, the contractions started. They were like menstrual cramps: annoying, but tolerable. We went out for dinner and I ate a ton! Then we went to get a video, and I commented at one point that I was actually fairly uncomfortable, to which Daniel replied, "If you're uncomfortable now . . . "

I told him not to finish that sentence, because he was voicing my fears exactly: if it hurt now, how was I going to survive later? I told him that what I needed from him, both now and in later labor, was reassurance and coaching. As a lifelong athlete, I respond well to encouragements like "Hang in there," "You're doing great," and so on. I didn't want patronizing remarks and I didn't want to be told what to do. Daniel agreed, but at that point he was still convinced that he'd merely irritated my cervix, and that this wasn't the real thing, despite the fact that the baby was due two days later.

We went home and watched the movie, more or less. I couldn't concentrate, so I tried to get some sleep. While flipping through the channels before turning off the tube, I came across a story on quin- and sextuplets. It certainly put everything in perspective.

I didn't get much sleep, what with mild diarrhea all night, and the contractions. At about 2:00 a.m. I got up, got my hot water bottle (my constant companion during years of menstrual cramps), sat in my rocker, timed contractions, and dozed. I put a garbage bag on the rocker beneath me so that if my water broke I wouldn't stain it. As the night wore on, the contractions became closer together and I mused on the fact that I might really be in labor and really be about to become a mother. It still seemed pretty abstract at that point. I dozed on and off in the chair, watching the clock and noticing that slowly but surely the contractions were coming closer together.

At about 6:30 a.m., the contractions had been three to five minutes apart for about an hour and a half. The midwife had told me to call her when the contractions were three minutes apart for two hours, so I

31

figured I'd give her a ring. Daniel, half-awake, told me that there was no way it was happening that fast. I said a call wouldn't hurt. The service asked me how far I lived from the hospital (10 minutes on a bad day), if I had been checked for dilation (no), and so on. They called back five minutes later and said, "Come on down." I relayed this message to Daniel, who wondered if he had time to take a shower. "Yes," I said, "but it had better be quick."

By now I needed to really focus during each contraction. They were becoming very intense and painful. They had the same cramplike quality as before, down low, but now they were more powerful—a tight, squeezing sensation. They are hard to describe, but they definitely took my breath away. The contractions were pretty regular at three minutes apart, although now that I'd been told to come into the hospital, I stopped paying much attention to the timing and began to focus on the fact that we were really going in.

In between contractions I was fine, but I could no longer walk or talk during one. I recall that after his shower, as Daniel called both sets of parents to let them know what was happening, I was kneeling, with one foot on the floor, the other on the couch, trying to breathe and to hurry him along. We left for the hospital around 7:45 a.m. and got there about 15 minutes later. As we walked toward admitting (I'm very macho—no wheelchair for me!), I turned to Daniel and said, "I still can't believe I'm having a baby!" and I wasn't kidding. I had loved being pregnant and had even taught aerobics two days before. But I never really thought I would have an actual *baby!* With all the significant milestones in my life, I've tended to believe that they only happen to other people, until they actually happen to me. So it was with having a baby. It just wasn't real until it really happened.

We were shown right to the Labor and Delivery room and I was hooked up to monitors for a while. I was checked for dilation before being put on the monitors, and Ruth, the midwife, told me I was 4 centimeters, and that she could push me to 5. I changed into a hospital "johnny." I had expected to wear my sweats and walk around a lot, but now I opted for the johnny and really only felt like sitting in the bed at that point, so I was happy to be on the monitors. After maybe a half hour, I was pretty uncomfortable and the nurse and midwife suggested that I get into the shower, which sounded good to me. I sat with the showerhead on my belly for a good two hours. Daniel checked in occasionally, but all I really wanted was to have my water bottle refilled periodically and to have him change the CDs on the portable player we had brought. I was really in a deep concentration zone and wanted minimal interference from anyone else.

All kinds of thoughts were going through my head. My friend Nancy, a stoic woman and mother of three, had commented before the birth of her third, "Labor really sucks." Now I knew what she meant. It really was painful. I was wondering why all of us had pushed so hard for natural childbirth. The old "knock me out, wake me when it's over" was sounding pretty good to me then. I thought of the woman, a former colleague of Daniel's, whom we had bumped into at admitting, who was there for a scheduled C-section. I was actually jealous of her at that point.

Toward the end of my time in the shower, while I was moaning and groaning aloud, I told Daniel that I needed something to help with the pain. The nurse gave me an injection right away. I was in the bed from then on, sitting up in a position that made me feel like Buddha, with the soles of my feet together and this big belly.

After the injection, I could relax between contractions, and I was having a much nicer time. I could hear Daniel and the nurse chatting about me, while I was sitting there, blissfully able to relax and to focus during the contractions. After about an hour and a half or so, the drug began to wear off. I requested another half-dose, which they gave me, but they told me that it probably wouldn't take as well as the first. They were right. The contractions were much closer together now, and at the peak of each one, I felt really nauseous. Just as I thought I was going to vomit, the contraction would subside, so I began to find the nausea reassuring because it meant the contraction was about to "break."

At this point, Wendy, the nurse, came in and told me that I had to decide whether I wanted my membranes ruptured. I asked why on earth I'd want that, since it would probably hurt more afterward. She told me it would speed things up. I said things were going quite fast enough, thank you. Ruth, the midwife, was checking my dilation right then and told me I was at 9 centimeters. That's when the membranes ruptured on their own.

Now the feeling of needing to push was growing. This was when the breathing techniques I had learned were really helpful. I was using the "ha-ha-hee" Lamaze breathing. It was only through intense focus that I was able to resist the urge to push. But it was growing stronger, and as it became overwhelming, I told Daniel to go find Wendy and Ruth (who were off arranging coverage for their other deliveries) because I couldn't *not* push.

When they all returned, Ruth told me I could push with the next contraction. I gave my first two pushes while semirecumbent, but then requested that they put up the squat bars. Instead, Ruth suggested kneeling on the bed, with my chest up against the raised head of the bed. I tried that and liked the position, so I stayed there.

I remember an overwhelming feeling of terror and very briefly thinking, "I can't do this!" Then Daniel stepped in and really helped me focus on my breathing, and particularly on taking cleansing breaths between the contractions. I seem to recall that, to avoid pushing at the wrong moment, I stated each time, "I'm going to push now." I also had so much faith in the strength of my muscles that I was sure each push would just send this baby flying out. After some pushing, the baby was on my pubic bone and it hurt. As I pushed, I was saying, "Get this baby out!" I didn't yell or scream, but I was quite insistent. I could feel the perineum stretching, which was very uncomfortable. I felt it burning, like I was going to split in half.

 I REMEMBER AN OVERWHELMING FEELING OF TERROR AND VERY BRIEFLY THINKING, "I CAN'T DO THIS!" THEN DANIEL STEPPED IN AND REALLY HELPED ME FOCUS ON MY BREATHING.

As the burning grew worse, Ruth asked me if I wanted to reach down and feel the head. I actually had to stop and think about this. I guess I didn't want to be distracted. I wanted to finish the job. But I did reach down and suddenly was transformed by the reality of it. There really was a head there, oh my goodness! This was amazing! I pushed again, then Daniel said, "Look at the *punum!*" (Yiddish for "face") and, thinking that meant it was a boy (because I don't know Yiddish), I said, "What is it?" He said, "I don't know, it's just the head." Then Ruth delivered the shoulders. I looked down and I said, "It's a girl! She's so little." I tried to pick her up while I was still kneeling, which was pretty clumsy. I commented that she was very slippery, so Ruth said they would clean her up a little. Then she was whisked to the warmer and I turned around and sat down. It was 2:11 p.m.

Miriam was handed back to me moments later wrapped in a blanket and I promptly forgot everything about the pain of the previous six hours. I was amazed by this tiny, pink creature and by the fact that we were really parents. Then I returned to my semirecumbent "Buddha" position and held Miriam while Ruth delivered the placenta. It happened pretty shortly after the delivery, but I wasn't really paying attention and it didn't hurt at all. I looked at the placenta, although I hadn't really planned to. I had a few small labial tears, but no cervical tears or tears of the perineal muscle. This is what I had aimed for by choosing first to squat and then to kneel during the pushing stage. Ruth did some minor repairs while I held Miriam and marveled over her. Daniel videotaped Miriam and me, and we made about a million phone calls, while Miriam quietly observed the world around her. I tried to get her to nurse immediately, but she wasn't the least bit interested, and in fact she didn't really nurse until the next day.

It's been nearly nine months since that day and I can't believe how the time has flown. I have fallen right into motherhood and I love it!

In fact, I have an overwhelming urge to get pregnant again, though I'm planning to wait for a little while. I'm sure next time I'm in labor, I'll be thinking "This sucks," but I know that immediately afterward I will be just as sure that it is worth it.

Interestingly, the experience has developed more intensity and depth in some ways as it recedes into the past. It's hard to be truly present in the miraculous moment with so much "sensory input" (i.e., pain), but as the pain fades, the mystery and miracle of childbirth fill in. Sometimes it's hard to believe I actually accomplished this feat, that Miriam grew inside me, and that I got her out, with her daddy's help.

They Call Him Lucky

Janet was 34 and director of sales for a Manhattan publisher when her son was born in a New York hospital via an emergency C-section. Her husband, Jeff, a composer, was also 34. They were living in Brooklyn at the time.

When I passed my due date, April 21, time began to move in slow motion. Seven days later, I had a checkup with my doctor. Everything looked fine, though it appeared I might be developing toxemia. My ankles had begun to swell, and my blood pressure was elevated, so my doctor scheduled a non-stress test for two days later—Friday, May 4. During the test, the baby had a somewhat irregular heartbeat and they found that my amniotic fluids were quite low. My doctor said that if I did not go into labor over the weekend, she would induce me on Monday.

I had a feeling I wouldn't make it to Monday, and sure enough, Sunday night, May 6, I lost my mucous plug. My husband and I were just sitting down to dinner at home when I felt very wet. I didn't think my water had broken, but I went to the bathroom to check. Based on everything I'd read, I guessed it was my mucous plug. It was very white. But I felt no discomfort at all, so we finished dinner and I went to bed at the usual time, 10:00 p.m.

At 2:00 a.m. on May 7, I was awakened by an extraordinarily painful contraction. It was bone-breaking pain, and as it turned out, the most painful contraction of my entire labor. It felt like someone had taken one of my vertebrae and broken it in half. I don't know why it was so painful, but I literally leapt out of bed. I immediately went downstairs and started making casseroles. I had a nesting instinct to make casseroles. I hadn't planned on this. I just felt compelled to do it.

The contractions were about five minutes apart from their outset. Though I knew this was the real thing, different from the less intense contractions I'd felt for the last few weeks, I felt it was too early to phone the hospital or wake my husband. Two hours later, when I finished cooking, at about 4:00 a.m., I went upstairs, took a very long shower, shaved the part of my legs I could reach, washed my hair, and made myself as beautiful as possible for the blessed event. Then I woke my husband.

I called my doctor at about 4:30 a.m. and was told to come to the hospital right away—I think she could tell by my voice that I was in pain. The contractions were really beginning to hurt. I was still breathing through them, but my voice was breaking, and I was scared. I am an asthmatic, and though I wasn't in distress, I was beginning to worry that I wouldn't be able to breathe through the labor (in the end I never had any problems with that).

My husband is terrified of hospitals. He was so anxious about going to the hospital, and upset because I was in pain, that he got lost trying to get us from Brooklyn to Manhattan, a trip we'd made a million times before. It took us an hour to get there and it should have taken 20 minutes. Finally, we arrived at the emergency room at about 6:00 a.m. The emergency room doctor who examined me found I was only 1 or 2 centimeters dilated, but my blood pressure was extremely elevated, a sign that I may have become affected by the toxemia, so he admitted me at once. I am usually quite calm, but now I couldn't stop crying. When the doctor asked me what was wrong, I remember saying that I was scared. And I was.

I went upstairs and began to labor in a private birthing room. Once I settled in, everything seemed manageable. My husband and I sat there holding hands.

My doctor arrived at 7:00 a.m. and began to monitor my labor. It made me feel calm just to have her around. If she had any concern about my high blood pressure, she didn't show it. She was, however, very concerned about the baby's irregular heartbeat.

I made no progress, so at 10:00 a.m., they broke my water. Because I was hardly dilated, this hurt a great deal, probably more than anything else in the labor. Still, nothing happened. I didn't dilate any more.

Around 11:00, my husband was told this would take a long time, and that he should go to lunch, so he did. As I continued to labor, the baby's heart rate kept dropping, indicating distress, and an internal fetal monitor was placed on the baby's head. Since I wasn't very dilated, still only about 2 centimeters, the insertion of the monitor was also extremely painful.

At about noon, I requested an epidural. The contractions were beginning to become more painful, and I was worried that if I didn't get the epidural started now, I would miss the window of opportunity when it was allowed and then not have it later when things were really painful. The anesthesiologist came immediately and the drip was started within 15 minutes of my request. As it turned out it was great that I had it in—it allowed Harry to be born as quickly as possible later.

THE NURSES LITERALLY PUSHED MY HUSBAND OUT OF THE WAY AND RAN WITH ME ON THE GURNEY TOWARD THE OPERATING ROOM.

A few minutes after the epidural kicked in, my husband returned from lunch and sat down with me. About 15 minutes later, the baby's heart rate dropped so far that my doctor suddenly said, "Janet, we're not doing this anymore. We are not going to wait. We are doing an emergency C-section."

My husband and I were both shocked, and we didn't have any time to react. The nurses literally pushed my husband out of the way and ran with me on the gurney toward the operating room. Jeff told me later that my doctor, who is an immensely calm, wonderful woman and mother of two, took him by the arm and showed him where to put on his gown and actually led him to the operating room. He felt that it was extraordinary that she would stop to show her concern for him in the middle of an emergency situation.

Our son was born seven minutes later. Jeff was sitting beside me at the head of the gurney with his head next to mine. He held my hand and looked into my face the entire time. He didn't watch the surgery. As she was delivering the baby, my doctor said, "Janet, I have never seen anything like this." The baby's umbilical cord was wrapped five times around his neck. (We found out later that he had such an extraordinarily long umbilical cord that the doctor sent it off for medical research.) This meant that with each contraction, his umbilical cord was being so compressed and crimped that he was almost completely cut off from his blood and oxygen supply, hence his distress.

Also, he had swallowed meconium and his lungs needed to be suctioned, so they were working on him for what seemed like about five minutes before they even told us whether we had a boy or a girl. We were terrified because we heard no sound and were too frightened to make a peep ourselves. Finally, we heard a cry, and we asked what we had. A boy! He weighed 6 pounds, 10 ounces and was 21 inches long.

While the neonatal team worked on the baby, the doctor had been stitching me up. Before she was finished, the minute Harry was given passing Apgar scores, he was handed to me, and placed at my neck, between my husband's face and mine. My husband and I both clearly remember him craning his little neck up to tilt his head and sniff me, and look me right in the face. All was well. We recognized each other!

The next day, I asked my doctor how long it would have been before Harry would have suffered brain damage. She replied, "Fourteen minutes—and we delivered him in seven!"

If I had had a choice, I never would have chosen a C-section. I took a long time to heal. And when it came time to deliver my daughter, I was adamant that I wanted to try to deliver vaginally (and I did!). But in the end, we were very, very grateful that our son was born healthy. After his birth, we nicknamed him "Lucky" after the puppy who was revived in *101 Dalmatians*. He's nine now and we *still* call him that.

All's Well That Ends Well

Ruth was 30 years old and her husband, Thomas, was 38 when their first child was born in a hospital in London. Thomas is a computer programmer, and Ruth is a scholar of Chinese history. Ruth's pregnancy was fine until she developed preeclampsia in the 34th week. She was admitted to the hospital for treatment, where she remained until her son was born two weeks later. Underscoring her practical response to the situation, her e-mail messages to me always ended with: Person-in-the-Street: Do you want a boy or a girl? Parent-to-Be: Yes!

The baby was due on August 6. When I went for my routine eight-month checkup on July 4, my midwife began by digging out the results of the previous week's blood tests for review. The results had been unsatisfactory, but that was no cause for concern in itself. Next she took my blood pressure. It had been rising gradually in the preceding weeks, and this day it finally reached an unacceptable level. Then my urine test revealed a high level of protein. The blood test results and the rising blood pressure were worrisome enough to

44

consider admitting me to the hospital, but the amount of protein in the urine was the final straw. The three factors combined were a strong indication of preeclampsia. At this point, my midwife said, "I'm going to phone my friend up at the hospital, 'cuz that's where you're going." When I asked her if I could ride my bike there, she firmly said, "No!" She asked if Thomas was able to go with me, but he'd finally gotten a job just a month before. At that moment, he was taking an exam and would be spending the rest of the week commuting to Surrey, south of London, every day for a course he was taking. My midwife said, "It's nothing to panic about . . . " so when I phoned my mum at work, I told her not to come.

Sensing trouble, I scooted back to my office and dashed off the one letter that really could not wait, before taking the bus to the hospital, where Mum showed up shortly afterward. By this time my blood pressure had spiked dramatically, so they gave me a "crunch"—a nasty-tasting orange blood pressure-lowering drug. The external monitor showed no problems with the baby, but nobody was about to let me go home because indeed I had preeclampsia, a high blood pressure condition that can deprive the fetus of nutrients. Thomas got home that evening to find phone messages from my mum, and he came to the hospital with my bag, which with lucky foresight I had packed the previous weekend.

There followed two whole weeks in the hospital, on blood pressure medication, having my blood pressure checked every four hours. Otherwise, I was fine. I had no other symptoms of hypertension except for a tiny bit of swelling in my ankles in the last few days.

It was one of the hottest Julys we've had in nearly 20 years. The hospital sits on the top of a hill and is one of those concrete and glass boxes that soaks up heat and has no place to send it. Like most buildings in Britain, it is not air-conditioned, as it rarely gets hot enough there to need it. The windows opened, but there was no breeze. The curtains were thin and didn't block much of the heat. It was hot!

The first week, I borrowed a laptop so I could do a bit of work, and I managed to hold a previously scheduled meeting, in the hospital, with a colleague. But boredom quickly became my main problem. There wasn't much to do. I had my work, and I could read, but the heat sapped my energy and made me less inclined to do anything that felt strenuous. I had little company, and nothing much was on television during the day. The second week in the hospital, I passed the time by watching the daytime soaps, trying to guess the plots.

By this time, numerous discussions with doctors had made it clear that while they would have liked to do it earlier, they would wait to induce me at week 37. There was more protein in my urine, so my condition was gradually deteriorating, but if we waited until 37 weeks, the baby would not be technically premature unless it was very small, which from the ultrasound seemed unlikely.

Thomas and I had to throw all our ideas about a natural childbirth out the window and accept that this was going to be a managed birth. We were disappointed, but we had tried to be realistic and practical throughout the pregnancy, so we were able to accept this and move forward. We repeatedly went over the procedures used to induce labor so that we would know what was happening when, and why, and so that we would understand everything. My caregivers were keen for me to have an epidural because that helps to keep the blood pressure down, and they made it clear that in the worst case scenario, we might even be talking about an emergency cesarean. If it came to that, it would be best to have the epidural already in place. I had a special meeting with an anesthetist to discuss the procedure and to reassure me about the concerns I had over an epidural causing back trouble later. (I already have a bad back and didn't want it made worse.) He told me there is no clear link at all between epidurals and back pain, and that it is much more likely that bad backs are a result of the physical exertions of motherhood rather than a side effect of epidurals. I still wanted to avoid an epidural if possible, but at least now I wasn't worried about it if I needed one.

My cervix was already very ripe on the Friday before my scheduled induction, and I was dilated 1 centimeter. Early Monday morning, July 17, a doctor stripped my membranes and we hoped it wouldn't take too much more to get my labor going. I had hardly slept the night before and was tired before we started. Thomas arrived at 6:00 a.m. and soon after, I had prostaglandin gel applied to my cervix as a mild, relatively noninvasive way of inducing labor. We spent the morning reading the papers and then started reading books. By lunchtime, nothing at all had happened. In the early afternoon, we took up residence in a delivery room (this one came with a wooden hospital bed and was one of only two rooms on the unit with a window). After settling into our room, we met our midwife, who was perfectly pleasant, but we didn't really click. I felt she didn't take much notice of what I was saying—not out of malice, just out of what I can only describe as absentmindedness or preoccupation. After the midwife left, a doctor came and broke my waters. This was most uncomfortable, and I was surprised by how hot the water was, not just warm as I had expected. After that I was encouraged to walk around some, which brought on a few mild contractions that reminded me of menstrual cramps. I put on my TENS machine, a device that delivers a small electrical pulse to the part of the body where you attach it. Applied to your back, it helps reduce the pain of the contractions. I also had a lavender footbath, which had no effect whatsoever, but was a nice thought anyway.

However, things were clearly going to go on for a long time with not a lot happening so the doctor put an IV needle in my arm and the midwife set up a Pitocin drip. Thomas and I wandered around a bit more while I tried to prepare myself mentally for labor.

Right up to the day of my induction, I had been hoping for a natural childbirth, and that my body would comply with my wishes. Having my cervix ripened and beginning to dilate the Friday before had fueled my hope, so although things were under way, I really wasn't ready mentally. It also did not help that, due to my early hospital admission, I hadn't completed the childbirth preparation classes. And the repeated explanations of what might happen had only prepared me for the worst, so I hadn't really given much thought to the possibilities for a happier outcome. I only knew I wasn't quite ready to have this baby! But I also knew I didn't have a choice anymore. That's how I resolved it. I realized that sometimes you do things because the moment is right, but sometimes you have to do things because it is time to, regardless of how you feel about it.

Once the drip was in, it didn't take so very much to get me going. I think the amount of Pitocin was rather high at first, but then they reduced it because my contractions were coming in very hard and fast, and hitting me right where I get pain when my back is acting up, only about ten times worse. At this point the TENS machine seemed largely ineffective, though I didn't have it turned up very far because I didn't like the way it buzzed. I said to Thomas, "I think I'm going to want an epidural." A short time afterward, I said, this time loudly and clearly, "I want an epidural," and silently added, "*Now!*" Thomas quickly relayed my demand.

This happened to coincide with the shift change. Our new midwife, Liz, was much younger and seemed more focused, while still being very nice, and I knew we'd get on fine. Both midwives were there for the insertion of the epidural. Having it put in wasn't much fun. You have to curl up on your side and hold completely still through one or two contractions while the needle is inserted, and the needle crunches and grates as it goes in. But once the drug took effect it was wonderful. Thomas and I sat on the bed and watched my contractions on the external monitor for perhaps three or four hours. Because I was a bit constipated I was offered the choice of an enema or suppositories. I should really have accepted them when they were first offered to me earlier. I took some suppositories but trying for what seemed like ages and ages, all I managed to pass was one suppository!

It was very quiet on the delivery suite (except for the yells of the women across the hall). At one point a different midwife took over so

Liz could have a break. Then, after all the waiting, suddenly everything seemed to happen at once. The epidural began to wear off, so it was re-dosed, but this time with no great effect. Liz examined me and said, "About 1 or 2 centimeters to go." Then a contraction came, the lip of cervix disappeared, and she said, "On the other hand, I think you're about ready to push." She suggested I might want to change my position. I had been sitting somewhat propped up, and she thought it would be much easier for me if I pushed on all fours, even though I had the epidural. I was glad the midwife suggested the move, as I never would have thought to raise the possibility. I assumed that with my IVs and the epidural in place, a needle might fall out somewhere, but I was wrong. The midwife didn't think changing position was unusual. Since midwives deliver the uncomplicated deliveries in Britain, I was com-fortable with her expertise, and due to my unpreparedness, I was also pretty reliant on her suggestions.

Meanwhile, Thomas sat next to me, feeding me ice chips, re-minding me to relax (which was invaluable), and putting the Entonox mouthpiece in my hand when the contractions came. (Entonox is a gas administered through a nose- and mouthpiece. You hold it to your face and can regulate the amount you want yourself. It is not generally used in the United States.) Thomas was wonderful. It all would have been much harder without him.

Pushing was excruciatingly painful, despite the epidural. I held back a bit on each push because the burning sensation in my perineum was so great and I really did not want to tear. I felt like I was trying to pass a huge watermelon. After about 45 minutes, I suddenly realized, after all our preparations for the worst, that this was going to be a normal delivery. Wow! Nobody had said anything about only letting me push for a certain length of time, but I knew there was a limit, and I was determined that nothing was going to stop me now. So I stopped holding back, pushed harder, and thought, "Damn the pain!" When the baby's head crowned, Liz asked my permission to apply a fetal scalp electrode, as the external monitor kept losing track of the heartbeat. Of course we said yes. It seemed that far too many contractions later (but probably not that many, really), out came the head. What a sensation of relief. Thomas said it looked really strange to see the baby's head sticking out of me, all funny colors and still not breathing.

The midsummer dawn had just barely begun breaking (it comes quite early at this latitude) and then there was what felt like the longest wait before the final contraction. Out came the rest of the baby at 2:39 a.m. on Tuesday, July 18. Liz had fetched back the midwife who'd relieved her so she could be there for the delivery, too, and the two of them caught the baby as it passed between my legs. They put him on the bed beneath me. I said, "It's a little boy!" and knelt over him with Thomas. I was just amazed and overcome with emotion. Thomas's face when he looked at Sam was so wonderful, so full of love. I will never forget that feeling. Liz asked Thomas if he wanted to cut the cord, and he was surprised at how tough it was. Then I sat down, leaned back, and held the baby while the placenta was delivered.

The baby weighed 6 pounds 3 ounces. We still hadn't decided on a name for a boy, so at that point he was nameless. He was a little cool so Liz fetched a warming lamp for him to lie under for a bit. I had a

1-centimeter, second-degree tear, which was stitched under local anesthesia with one internal, dissolving stitch and one external, silk stitch. (Apparently the midwives all use silk for the external stitches, whereas doctors use catgut, which, I'm informed, feels like barbed wire after a couple of days!) An auxiliary nurse came and gave me a bed bath, and finally the three of us were left alone for a bit. We were all so worn out that we went right to sleep!

Later, after seeing me back to my room, Thomas went home, phoned his mum in Australia, and then slept. I gave him the final say over names, and in the evening he came back with my mum. I was to stay in the hospital for at least five days to keep an eye on my blood pressure, and ended up staying even longer because of feeding problems with the baby, but that, as they say, is another story . . .

The epidural was great. I'll still try to do without it next time, because I hope that I'll have a chance to get used to the contractions before they get really big.

Next time I also want to make sure they let the cord stop pulsating before it is cut. (I don't know if they did or not this time.) And if the baby needs to be warmed up, I'll ask if I can cuddle him to me rather than using a lamp.

Eighth in a Line of Firstborn Sons

*Nina, a Swedish woman, delivered her first baby in a
Florida hospital when she was 29 years old. At the time
she was working as a translator and personnel director at a
linguistics software company, and as an aerobics instructor.
Her husband, Patrick, 35, was a CPA. They live on an
island off the coast of Southwest Florida.*

Sunday, August 1, 1993 was a very hot, humid, and sunny afternoon. My husband and I decided to go down to the beach, where we met our neighbors. We were sitting in the sun for a while, talking and having a good time, and then my neighbor and I decided to go into the water. After a few minutes, I started feeling contractions. It felt like a tightening around the stomach and some pressure on my pelvic bone.

The Thursday before, I had been at the doctor's office. At that time I was 2 centimeters dilated and the baby's head was already very far down. The doctor could actually touch the baby's head. He told me

53

that the baby had hair, and also that he didn't think I would go over the weekend.

In a previous surgery, some of my cervix had been removed. Because of this, it was abnormally thin, and it has some scar tissue. The doctor said this would not affect my delivery, but that my dilation might stall, as it apparently had, at about 2 centimeters. Then, once it started to dilate again, it would open very quickly.

We decided to leave the beach after only an hour, even though my contractions were irregular.

But what bad luck! When we got home we discovered that of all days, this was the one our air conditioner broke down. It was about 100 degrees in our house. I started to freak out, walking through the house saying, "I can't believe this is the day the stupid air conditioner decides to break down!" That was not a lot of fun. I took a shower, and when I got out of the shower and started trying to put some clothes on, I was already sweating again and freaking out.

The contractions were actually far apart, maybe half an hour between each, so we decided that I should go to my in-laws' condominium nearby, where I could be in their air-conditioning while my husband tried to fix ours, so I went there. But first, of course, I had to cry in the driveway. My husband wanted me to calm down before I went, so I sat and cried in the driveway for about 10 minutes. Then I realized that crying wasn't going to help, so I calmed down, and then I drove to my in-laws'.

My husband's parents hadn't been staying in the condo for several months. So when I walked in, I was met by this terrible, moldy smell. It's the kind of moment you don't appreciate too much. But at least it was cool. I sat there with open windows and with the air conditioner running for about two hours, napping for a little while. The contractions were almost gone now. Then my husband called me. He had fixed our air conditioner and I could go back home, which was much better.

At home, I lay down. Later on, my neighbors called and asked if we wanted to come over for dinner, which was very nice of them since I certainly didn't feel like cooking that night. By this time, the contractions had pretty much stopped, so we went over to our neighbors and had dinner. We had some pasta and vegetables and I probably ate about 20 chocolate chip cookies. After the stomachache that followed, I will never eat another chocolate chip cookie . . . well, I guess that's not true.

We were playing cards and having a good time. About 9:00, my neighbor and I went for a walk with her dog, and my husband went home to do some work. I got home about 9:30.

As I was getting ready for bed I could still feel a few contractions, but they were not very strong and they were very far apart, so I didn't even time them. I sat down on the toilet and I did my thing, and then some more water came, eight ounces maybe. So of course I said, "Hmmm. What is this?" And then I started thinking, "Ahhhhh, this is it!" I said to my husband, "I think my water just broke." And he said, "You're kidding me!" He got really excited, and anxious, too. I called the doctor. The doctor on call was not my doctor, but he said he would call my doctor right away and let him know. He told me to go to the hospital right away. Because of my unusually thin cervix, and the fact that we lived on an island with a 30-minute drive ahead of us, he wanted us to be on our way.

Of course I wanted to first take a shower and shave and do all those important things you need to do before you go to the hospital. I was in the shower, shaving away, and my husband was standing at the front door with my bag, jumping up and down, screaming at me, "Hurry up! Hurry up! Hurry up!" He didn't want to waste any time, and he certainly didn't want me to have the baby in the car. But I was getting ready, and, of course, having problems deciding what to wear.

My water had broken at about 10:00 p.m., and it was about 10:30 or 10:45 by the time we finally left for the hospital. I was going through my list, making sure I had everything with me. I didn't have those very important sugar-free candies I wanted to suck on for energy, so I told my husband that we'd have to stop at the gas station and get some Certs or something. He said, "No way. We're not stopping anywhere. I'm going straight to the hospital. Once we are there, we can get them." I said, "Oh, please, please, please." My contractions were five minutes apart, and they were not strong. I was not very uncomfortable and I really wanted to have those Certs. I made him stop, and he ran in and got them, and came back and said, "Okay, now we're not stopping anywhere." He drove straight to the hospital and we were there by about 11:10 p.m.

Since I had pre-registered, signing in wasn't a big deal and I got in right away. All the papers were fine. They put me in a wheelchair and wheeled me right up to the maternity ward. We were only the second couple there that night, so we got one of the birthing rooms. One of the advantages of the birthing room is that you stay in the whole time until after you have the baby instead of having to be moved from a labor room to a delivery room. After the birth, you move to the maternity ward to a room that you share with one person. The suite had a rocking chair, a swivel chair, a television, and a birthing bed (they can take the bottom off of it when it comes time for pushing). You never have to move around, which I found was very comfortable. You also had your own bathroom to use whenever you wanted to.

Now it was about 11:25 p.m. and I was all set. I had my "pretty" gown on and everything, so my husband and I started walking around the maternity ward. We did about two or three laps, about 100 yards each, and then my contractions started to get really bad. That happened pretty quickly—they'd been pretty mild in the car. After arriving at the hospital, the contractions started to make me a bit more uncomfortable: they were about five, or maybe four minutes apart at that time. Now after walking for about 15 minutes, they were three minutes apart and they were really strong. It felt like they lasted forever, kind of overlapping each other. I had terrible pain and pressure on my pelvic bone. I felt like my whole insides were going to fall out. At the end, I was actually doubled over with pain and I couldn't walk anymore, so I half-crawled back to the birthing room and lay down in the bed there. I was in a lot of pain. By now I would say the contractions were about three minutes apart but I didn't have any relief between them, because the baby's head was so far down it created a terrible pressure on my pelvic bone. I didn't know what to do. I wanted to turn the time back about nine months.

People tell you labor pains are bad, but you can't describe just how bad they really are. I was trying to relax by taking slow, deep breaths, but I just couldn't handle it. The worst thing about it was that the pain never stopped.

I had pre-registered for the epidural in case it was needed, though seeing the needle in a childbirth education class made me quite afraid of it. But by the time I went into labor, I had seen it three times, in films and at the doctor's office, so at least it was familiar to me.

By about midnight, I couldn't handle the pain anymore. I was worried about how much worse it would get. I knew there were other drugs available, but that they might not be effective quickly enough for me, so I asked for the epidural. After the longest half-hour ever, the anesthesiologist finally came and at about 12:45, he gave me the epidural. I thought I would be very scared when they stuck the long needle into my spine, but compared to the pain from the contractions, I didn't care. As far as I was concerned they could do whatever they wanted as long as it took the pain away. As it turned out, the needle didn't bother me at all, and about 10 minutes after I got the epidural it started to work, and it was the most wonderful thing.

Right before I had the epidural I had such bad pains, my leg muscles had started cramping up on me and I was having spasms. My husband was trying to get me to relax. Of course he was doing the wrong kind of breathing, or what I thought at this point was the wrong kind of breathing, "Hee-hee-hoo! Hee-hee-hoo!" He was trying to be helpful, remembering the Lamaze class, standing there telling me, "Breathe like this," and I was saying, "Shut up! *You* breathe!" I didn't want to hear anything about breathing. I felt I was lucky to breathe at all. I was trying to relax with deep breathing and I just couldn't do it. But after I got the epidural, it was totally different. I could still feel the contractions, but they weren't painful anymore.

When I arrived at the hospital, I was 2 centimeters dilated; right before I got the epidural, I was 3 centimeters and then they didn't check me

for a while. Then, about 3:00 or 3:30 a.m., I started to feel the pain again. It was not as painful as before, but it definitely wasn't comfortable anymore, so I called the nurse. When she checked me, she said I was dilated 8 centimeters, and added, "We'd better call the doctor." Until this time, between 1:00 and 3:00 in the morning, my husband and I were both nodding off and we got some rest. I think that helped a lot, too, because then I had some strength when it came time to start pushing.

At about 4:00 the doctor came and checked me. I was 9 centimeters, so I had

MY HUSBAND WAS TRYING TO BE HELPFUL, STANDING THERE TELLING ME, "BREATHE LIKE THIS," AND I WAS SAYING, "SHUT UP! *YOU* BREATHE!"

to wait a bit longer. By about 4:45, I was fully dilated and it was time to start pushing. I had a wonderful nurse with me who helped me a lot by coaching me and saying how far out the baby was. This was good because at first I felt like I was pushing and pushing and nothing was happening. I couldn't really feel the baby moving, so she had to convince me that the baby was really coming. Then I figured it was worth it, and I kept on pushing. At about 5:10, they started getting excited, telling me I didn't have very long left. The nurse was holding my right leg, and my husband was holding my left leg. My feet were against their shoulders, and every time I had a contraction, they held my legs up so I could push against their weight and get some support. The baby was coming out more and more, and the doctor was saying, "Okay, now it's going to be one more push." So I was pushing really, really hard, and the baby didn't come out all the way, so the doctor decided to do an episiotomy.

My husband, who was holding my left leg, almost fainted when the doctor made the cut. When that contraction was over, my husband was still holding my leg up and I had to ask him to please let go. I think he was just holding onto something, anything, so he wouldn't fall over. The nurse asked him if he was okay. He said, "I think I'm fainting." This was not the best time for him to do that. Not a great support. The nurse told him to sit down and put his head between his legs.

Now it really was time for me to do the last push. They told me to push again, that this would be the last time, and that the head was coming out—and now I could feel it all. I felt something slippery coming out, and the stretching and burning finally stopped. I felt great! Excited! My husband looked up, and he saw the head come out. Then I had to stop while they made sure that everything was in the proper position.

For the last push, when the baby's body actually came out, my husband was still sitting down in his chair on the left side of the bed, and the baby was turned to the left, so he was the first one who could see that it was a boy. He started jumping up and down, screaming, "It's a boy! It's a boy!" He was very, very excited. My new son became the eighth in a line of firstborn sons in my husband's family, all named Patrick. So we immediately knew our baby's name: Patrick.

The first thing the doctor did was cut the cord. Then he attached the little clamp, wrapped the baby in a blanket, and put him on my breast, so I could start breastfeeding him right away. It was the most wonderful thing that had ever happened to me. I can't describe it. It was so emotional. I was just so very happy. I was exhausted, but so happy. I finally got to meet this little one who had been inside me for nine months whom I'd been wondering about.

During one of his first checkups, they discovered that our son had some heart irregularities, so he had to be kept on a monitor for the first day in the hospital. He had to have some tests, but whenever he was hungry, they brought him to me so I could breastfeed him. The tests all showed that nothing was wrong with him. That was a wonderful relief.

Just after the baby was born, before the epidural wore off, I felt really good. My husband and I started calling everybody telling them that the baby was born even though it was 6:00 in the morning. I called my Mom and my sister, and my brother in Sweden, and they were all excited.

They let you recover for a while in the birthing room, which was good. They helped me to the bathroom and made sure I was okay. Then they transferred me to the other room. At first, I was alone in the room and that was great. My legs were still a little numb, but I managed to take a shower. They brought my breakfast, but I was too excited to eat, so my husband ate it.

Shortly after we made all the calls to our families, my husband had to go home to meet the delivery people who were bringing the carpet for the baby's room at 8:30 that morning. Later my husband told me that on the drive home, he finally felt what had happened to him: he had become a father. And that made him think back to what his father's experience must have been like when he was born 35 years ago. Connecting their experiences brought tears to his eyes and made him feel proud. After meeting the delivery people, my husband came back to spend time with his new family.

About 9:00 a.m., the epidural started to wear off and then it wasn't as much fun anymore. I started to get really sore, and it was very hard to move around.

The hospital is not a good place to get any rest. Every couple of hours, they come in and check your temperature and your blood pressure, and in between that, you're just so sore, you can't really get comfortable. And the baby is being brought in every couple of hours because he's hungry. Then, if you drop off to sleep, your roommate wakes you because she's going to the bathroom, or doing something else. So, even though I was exhausted, I didn't get any sleep.

But we stayed in the hospital for two days, until my son was declared healthy. Then we came home to begin our new life.

At Home in the City

*Rachel, who delivered her baby at home with the help of a
midwife, a doula, and her husband, Duncan, 49, writes,
"I think it's helpful to know who I am (or at least who I was
when my daughter was born). I was almost 35 years old, quite fat
(5' 8" tall, 250 pounds before my pregnancy weight gain), and a
lawyer working in commercial litigation in a medium-size New York
City law firm. On the face of it, I was not an ideal candidate for
a home birth, because my weight and my age made me a
somewhat riskier patient than the ideal, which I imagined to be
a fit 25-year-old. Also, my profession might have scared some
practitioners who were worried about malpractice suits."*

The idea of a home birth had been brewing in my head for a long time. For me a home birth offered the benefits of being in control, being in familiar surroundings, and knowing that unnecessary medical interventions were not waiting for me in the operating room down the hall. But initially, the usual fears about what if

something went wrong and I couldn't get to the hospital on time got
the best of me, so I started with a hospital-based midwifery practice, on
the theory that I would get the best of both worlds that way.

However, during my fifth month, I went on the hospital maternity
ward tour and was turned off by the idea of having my baby there. The
birthing center in Manhattan, another alternative, had a hospital transfer rate of about 20 percent, and in my view, they were too rigid and for-
mulaic in their transfer policies. If your water breaks and you don't start
laboring within 24 hours, you are transferred, for example. It also didn't
help that every lawyer I knew in New York who had a baby, had had it
by C-section. I didn't want some hospital's inordinate concern about a
malpractice suit landing me on the operating table. I quickly found a
midwife in New York City who did home deliveries and signed up with
her practice. Her office was even close to my apartment.

My entire pregnancy was uneventful. I think being fat actually
helped me in some ways. My size didn't change as much proportion-
ately as a slender woman's does, so I had fewer problems with body image and with the mechanics of moving the bulk of a pregnant body
around. My midwife was vigilant for any signs of an increase in blood
pressure or gestational diabetes, but neither of these risks from obesity
in pregnancy showed up.

I was due Tuesday, June 2, 1992, and I kept working right up to the
Friday before. Then I waited. And waited. The midwife was seeing me
pretty frequently, but neither the baby nor my cervix showed any signs
of being ready. This is one of the many places where I think the home
birth/midwifery choice saved me from unnecessary medical interven-

tions. In many obstetrical practices, I probably wouldn't have been "allowed" to go so far past my due date without being induced, despite my unripe cervix. Also, the midwife wasn't in a panic over the size of the baby even though it was late.

Finally, early on Wednesday morning, June 10, I started to have irregular but frequent, and painful, contractions. They felt like a belt tightening around my middle, while someone stabbed me in the center of my lower back. They were pretty consistent, and much worse than any menstrual cramps I'd ever had, and I've had some doozies.

This went on for three days. I would get two or three contractions that seemed to increase in length and in frequency. Then there would be a few longer gaps, and then sometimes a really long gap (about 20 minutes). Then the cycle would repeat. I was jumping out of my skin from the stress of timing contractions, and from constantly thinking "This is it!" and then, "No, this isn't it, yet." Then, "Well, this must really be it." You get the idea. By Friday, I was getting pretty hysterical from lack of rest and from the constant cycle of anticipation and disappointment, so the midwife called in the back-up obstetrician to get me a prescription for a sedative. That was a brilliant move, because Friday night's sleep was the last I got until after Hannah was born on Sunday afternoon.

Late Saturday evening, my husband and I were trying to distract ourselves by watching a funny movie on the VCR. We kept stopping the tape so he could press my back through the contractions. We were sitting on the sofa. Duncan was grinding his fists right into the center of my lower back, where the pain was the worst. Finally, we realized that the contractions were starting to increase in both frequency and length. We timed an hour of contractions, then called our doula and our midwife. The doula was about two hours away at a family reunion, so she sent her partner, who lived around the corner from us.

When the midwife arrived, thinking back on the days of false labor with no progression, I joked: "If I'm not at least 5 centimeters dilated, I'm gonna kill myself." She checked me and said, "Six centimeters. I guess you'll just have to live," and I whooped with glee.

I DEALT WITH THE PAIN BY FOCUSING MY ENERGY INWARD, TRYING TO WORK WITH THE PAIN INSTEAD OF AGAINST IT, AND WHEN THAT DIDN'T WORK, I JUST BELLOWED.

The pain in my back during the contractions was really awful. Hannah was posterior, with her back against mine, which meant that every contraction pressed her little bony spine right down on my spine. That hurt! I dealt with the pain by focusing my energy inward, trying to work with the pain instead of against it, and when that didn't work, I just bellowed: long, low-pitched groans. I was really loud. It felt like a deep internal pressure on the bones in my back and pelvis. If I felt that safe pain relief had been available, I would have taken it in a hot minute.

The doula was really helpful. I wasn't interested in food, so she made sure I had things to drink. She fixed snacks for my husband, pressed and kneaded my back, and said lots of soothing, encouraging things to me. When the other doula arrived a few hours later, I thought that her partner would leave, but they both decided to stay, out of the kindness of their hearts. I really felt like a queen bee, with two doulas, a midwife, and my husband all trying to make the birthing easier on me. My husband, who is 14 years older than me, and a bit compulsive about getting his sleep, was especially grateful for the doula's presence, since it gave him a chance to steal away from the scene for a catnap in the wee hours.

As Sunday's dawn broke over our tiny Manhattan garden, I waddled over to the sliding glass door to watch the sun come up over the buildings. The fresh morning air revived me a little. I'm afraid I don't remember the details of most of the last eight hours of my labor. It is a blur to me now. However, at that point, I still had a long way to go.

I continued to labor, progressing ever so slowly, less than a centimeter every two hours. I vomited and started feeling a little desperate at some time late in the morning, but I don't have a clue when I entered transition. I do remember at some point the midwife telling me I should lie down. I resisted, because my contractions felt worse when I was lying down, but she convinced me that they felt worse because they were more productive in that position. After I was lying down on the bed for about an hour, I finally made it from 8 to 9+ centimeters.

At about noon, the midwife told me that I had been stuck at 9 centimeters for a while. She explained that all that was left of the cervix was a little "lip" on one side. She told me that she could push the lip aside with her finger, and that this would probably get me pretty quickly to the second stage of labor. She also told me that it would hurt, a lot, and that she had to do it at the peak of a contraction. At this point, I was lying down on my bed, my hips elevated on a couple of

pillows to aid the midwife in getting a good view of what she was doing. She wasn't lying about the pain! The few seconds it took for her to
perform that procedure were the worst of the whole process. However,
I very soon felt the urge to push, so she was right to do it.

I had decided in advance that I wanted to birth in a semistanding
position. My thinking was that I didn't have strong enough leg muscles
to do a real squat, which looked to me like the fastest way to have a baby,
so semistanding seemed like the next-best option. I got up and stood at
the foot of my bed. I didn't realize it at the time, but I was balancing some
of my weight on the sharp edge of the front of the wooden platform with
my knees, which had a line of bruises on them for a week afterward from
the pressure. The doula and my husband helped me support my weight
as I stood, with my knees bent, bearing down on each contraction.

After 40 minutes or so, Hannah crowned. I felt a burning sensation
around my labia, and the midwife told me to try to breathe through a
contraction or two to slow down the baby and prevent tearing. Well,
the very next contraction was irresistible: I just couldn't help pushing.
Hannah came out all at once. She never turned, never was half-in, half-
out. She was just—schloop—there! It was 2:35 p.m., about 15 hours
after we had started timing contractions. Of course, if you count the
first three days of contractions it was much longer labor . . . but I don't.
Those contractions were unpleasant, but to me they weren't real labor.

The midwife caught Hannah, told me to lie down on the bed,
and handed her to me. I held her on my chest and looked her over. I
can honestly say my primary emotion was relief that the labor was over.
I really wasn't that interested in her for a few minutes. She wasn't

breathing right away, but the cord was giving her oxygenated blood, so there was no big rush or emergency. The midwife gently suctioned Hannah's throat. She coughed once or twice and then started breathing. It was all very calm. Hannah soon latched on for a nursing.

About 5 to 10 minutes after Hannah emerged, the midwife tied off her cord. Then Duncan did the actual cutting. I don't remember when exactly the placenta came. Hannah had latched on for her first nursing, and I think she stimulated a couple of contractions big enough to help me push out the placenta. I had torn some and did need some stitches, but the tear was very superficial and no muscle tissue was involved. Through all this, Duncan was stroking my hair, looking at Hannah, and saying, "Wow!"

HONESTLY, MY PRIMARY EMOTION WAS RELIEF THAT THE LABOR WAS OVER.

The midwife gave Hannah a bath, right on the bed, while the doulas cleaned up the mess. My husband's best friend arrived and shot a few minutes of videotape, then he and Duncan went out into the yard to bury the placenta under the dogwood tree. We spent the rest of the day relaxing; we ordered in some food and called our relatives.

All in all, I would say that home birth was the best option for me. I was not "brave." It was my fear of the hospital that drove me to do it. The only thing I wish had been different is that I had had some option for safe pain relief at home. I think I would like to try acupuncture, if I should ever have another baby.

The Epidural Was My Ticket

Leeann was 35 years old and a third-grade teacher when her daughter was born in a hospital in La Grange Park, Illinois. She has a neurological condition that required her to have as stress-free a labor and delivery as possible, so she decided to have an early epidural. Her husband, Steve, 32, was a computer programmer.

When I first told my third graders I was pregnant, one girl asked, "You're not going to drop that baby during math class, are you?" I assured her that it took a long time and a lot of work for babies to be born. Little did I know. As it turned out, my pregnancy was far more challenging than my labor.

During my first trimester, I had started seeing a high-risk obstetrician. I have a neurological condition known as Basilar migraines. A Basilar attack is not a headache, though a headache can sometimes accompany an attack. Rather, the attack causes the muscles in my body to freeze up; nothing moves, not even my eye or mouth muscles. The attack begins in my extremities and then moves toward my torso and head. After about 30 minutes, some movement is restored, but I need to sleep for a couple of hours before I am recovered.

An attack can be triggered by strenuous exercise, poor diet, or excessive heat. At first, my husband and I were told we shouldn't have children, but after going to the Mayo and Loyola Clinics, we were convinced it would be safe for us as long as it was before I turned 35. The doctor felt that since other risk factors increased after that age, we might as well avoid them if we could. Her reasoning was that I already had enough risk factors without adding any more. Well, we were both lucky and surprised when we conceived the first time we tried. I was 34 years old.

During the pregnancy, I had to be hospitalized several times to receive intravenous rehydration because my first-trimester nausea was so severe. And in the eighth month, I had a severe Basilar attack, again requiring hospitalization. Since these attacks can be brought on by physical stress, we decided in advance that an epidural was warranted. It would keep me relaxed and relieve some of the stress of labor.

I met with an anesthesiologist at the hospital several weeks before the birth so he could examine me briefly and ask some questions. For example, we discussed the possibility of an emergency C-section, and he looked down my throat in case a breathing tube needed to be inserted quickly. Thankfully, neither was necessary, but I was pleased to know how thorough the doctor was.

I also paid close attention to the discussion of epidurals during our childbirth classes. The instructors taught us what happens to the body when an epidural is administered, as well as how and where the needle is inserted.

My pregnancy was challenging for yet another reason. I started having Braxton Hicks contractions in my seventh month. This excited me, as I figured my body was preparing for the birth and perhaps getting "in shape." By 35 weeks gestation, my doctors were saying I should have my bag packed. At 36 weeks, the baby's head was engaged. At 37 weeks, they told me to expect it any day. I was having contractions daily, some hard enough that I began wondering if I really would "drop the baby during math class"!

During that 37th week, we held an hour and a half parents' open house during which I introduced the teacher who was taking over my class. It was March, the middle of spring semester. While the parents were reviewing the children's work and talking to the new teacher, I was timing contractions. I was sitting down, so they probably thought I was just tired after teaching all day. Little did they know; I could not have stood up if I had to.

The new teacher and I planned to work together that week so the children would have a smooth transition between teachers, but the truth was, neither of us expected me to be there past that night. However, a pattern developed over the next two weeks, in which after several hours of contractions 7 to 10 minutes apart, they stopped. I actually worked with the new teacher through the end of the week as planned. Many times each day, I would time contractions while trying to concentrate very hard on what I was teaching. On Friday, I said my good-byes to friends, colleagues, parents, and students.

The following week, week 38, I waited and timed and waited. Contractions woke me up at night, but after a while, I got used to them—

sort of. Every time I went to the doctor for a checkup, I was told, "Any day now!"

On March 6, during week 39, I started timing contractions early in the morning. My husband left for work as usual (quite sure this was going to go on for several more weeks). After the contractions were six minutes apart for an hour, I called the doctor. She said to go to the hospital.

My husband had just arrived at work, so he caught the next train home and arrived an hour and a half later. Ten minutes before he walked through the door, the contractions stopped. Of course.

After waiting an hour, we called the hospital to let them know we weren't coming in after all. They advised us to go walking. So walk we did. For four and a half hours we walked a couple of malls. We were both exhausted. That night, three hours after I went to bed, the contractions began again. I slipped downstairs to watch television and to

THE BIRTH INSTRUCTOR HAD TOLD US IN CLASS THAT A SHOWER MIGHT EASE THE PAIN. WRONG!

start timing. After an hour, I took a shower. I remembered that the birth instructor had told us in class that this might ease some of the pain. Wrong! I leaned against the shower wall and thought to myself, Wow, I'm definitely in labor. I was surprised that the shower did not relax me, and in fact, it even seemed to increase my pain. In retrospect, I realize that my labor was progressing while I happened to be in the shower.

Straight out of the shower, I woke Steve and told him I needed him. He started timing contractions and I tried watching some stupid

4:00 a.m. infomercial. I was trying to breathe through the contractions and I was excited by my baby's pending birth. During an especially painful contraction, my husband said, "Breathe!" Enunciating very clearly, I informed him, "I *am* breathing!" (I wasn't.)

By 6:00 a.m., I was no longer worried they would send us home if we went to the hospital. The contractions were now no more than six minutes apart and were lasting at least 45 seconds. Steve was less convinced. In our relationship, we tend to discuss decisions extensively, and sometimes overanalyze them. This time, I insisted! I told him I wanted to go, and now. But first Steve took a shower, walked the dog, took the garbage out, and then, at last, put the bags in the car. Though I still had a grain of doubt that this was finally, really happening, I was not too happy about this wait. That half-hour seemed like an eternity.

We drove through snowy rain, and when we arrived at the hospital, Steve went inside, got a wheelchair, wheeled me to the check-in area, and then went back out to park our car. While I was giving answers to the clerk, I had several contractions. The admitting officer called for someone to take me to Labor and Delivery immediately. No one came, and three minutes later, I had another contraction. Then another. Despite the roomful of people waiting to be admitted, the officer told her supervisor she was wheeling me upstairs herself because she had no intention of delivering this baby.

Steve caught up with us on the way to the Labor and Delivery room. Upon examination, I was fully effaced and 4 centimeters dilated. The anesthesiologist was busy, so they gave me a shot of morphine, a drug chosen because of my Basilar migraine condition, so I could relax while I waited.

Finally, the anesthesiologist arrived to insert the epidural. The entire procedure took only 15 minutes. He cleaned an area on my back with what felt like alcohol, tore pieces of tape and stuck them to the metal sides of the bed (this seemed to take most of the time), prepared the needle (which I didn't see because my back was to him), fingered my spine, and then inserted the needle while I tried not to move. That was the hardest part—leaning over and not moving during the contractions, which were coming every two or three minutes now. The needle went in on the first try, and I soon got used to being careful of the tape on my back, which held the needle in place.

After the epidural took effect, I napped, chatted, and relaxed. I had a "high" epidural, which is one that numbed me fairly far up my torso, so I felt no pain at all during labor. I never felt out of control. I was mostly calm and peaceful as we progressed from one stage of labor to the next. Steve was with me the entire time. When I napped, he did some work on his laptop. When I was awake, he put on music for me, and we chatted.

At 1:00 p.m., they got the room prepared for birth. I was more upright now, leaning against Steve. A few minutes before 2:00 p.m., I started pushing. Despite the epidural, I felt a slight urge to push, and someone touched my perineum to help me visualize where to push, but otherwise, I felt nothing.

I had on an internal monitor, and, suddenly, we saw that the baby's heart rate was dropping and staying down for too long after the contractions. The doctor decided to help the baby along with a vacuum extractor, which looks something like a plunger. The doctor performed an episiotomy, and during a push, attached the suction cup to the baby's head, then guided the extractor and baby. At one point the doctor asked me to stop pushing as she unwrapped the cord from around the baby's shoulder. Because the cord was around the baby's shoulder, as I pushed, it was getting pinched against my bones, causing her decelerated heartrate.

 ONCE THE HEAD AND SHOULDERS WERE DELIVERED, I GOT TO PULL HER OUT THE REST OF THE WAY. THAT WAS AN AWSOME EXPERIENCE!

Once the head and shoulders were safely delivered, I got to pull Emma Ann the rest of the way. At 2:22 p.m., she slid into the world with eyes open wide. Pulling this slippery, warm, wet person out of my body was an awesome experience! At that point, Steve tried to see between her legs and said, "It's a boy!" The doctor said, "You might want to look again . . . " Steve had seen the umbilical cord wrapped through her legs as I was pulling her out and up onto my stomach! Our little climber crawled up to my chest and looked straight into my eyes. I fell in love immediately. Our daughter was born. Steve, with shaking hands, cut the cord. Later, he said he felt a mixture of excitement, fear, and surprise that the cord, which looked easy to cut, was much stronger and more difficult to cut than he expected.

I am so thankful that an epidural was available to me, because I believe it was what allowed me the privilege of welcoming my child into the world and caressing her in my arms immediately. I'd been waiting for that moment since I was a young girl. My biggest fear had been that I would have an attack and then have to have a C-section. Granted, this would not have been the end of the world, and I would have had a wonderful, healthy child either way, but I really did want to give birth without the negative experience of having a Basilar spell. While the epidural obviously couldn't take away the work, the exercise my body was doing, it did keep me breathing regularly and minimized the stress. So for me, the epidural was my ticket to a safe vaginal birth.

LUCAS'S BIRTH

Rewards of Research

*Pam and Jerry live near Nashville, Tennessee. Their first child
was born in a hospital when Pam was 34 years old and Jerry
was 35. She is a manufacturing engineer, and her husband
is a finance manager. Pam and Jerry thoroughly researched
their options and then wrote a birth plan that was
approved by their obstetrician and pediatrician.
Happily, all went according to plan.*

When I became pregnant I knew very little about pregnancy and childbirth, but I am the type who always tries to learn as much as I can about something when it becomes important to me. A friend at work gave me some literature on the Bradley method of natural childbirth, and what I read made so much sense to me that I signed us up for the 10-week class. The Bradley class, eating right, keeping active, doing pregnancy exercises, reading the pregnancy and breastfeeding books all helped me feel more confident.

But it was only gradually that I came to realize that in the pregnancy and childbirth arena, I was the customer. I felt I could and should be the one influencing the situation. Once we learned what was standard procedure in the hospital of our choice and compared that to the many other possibilities for a birth experience, we realized we had to take control in order to get what we wanted. We drafted a birth plan and arranged an office visit with our primary obstetrician so we could review our plan together, to see where we differed from their recommendations. I'm afraid the doctor's office labeled us as "pests," but we did get them to agree to our plan.

I CAME TO REALIZE THAT IN THE PREGNANCY AND CHILDBIRTH ARENA, I WAS THE CUSTOMER.

We also researched the care of our new baby. We were surprised to learn that in this state, following a hospital birth the primary care of the newborn immediately transfers from the obstetrician to the pediatrician. I had thought the obstetrician would be in charge of both mother and baby until our discharge from the hospital. So we searched for and found a pediatrician who supported our desire to keep our baby with us for the first precious hours after birth. As long as the baby was healthy, we didn't want those alert hours spent with hospital staff weighing, measuring, bathing, and treating the baby with eye drops, when instead we could be establishing the breastfeeding relationship and bonding with one another.

On Friday, May 1, 1992, three days past my due date, something woke me up at 2:30 a.m., and I felt an intense urge to run to the toilet.

As I navigated the short distance between our bed and the bathroom, I felt a gush. By "holding," I managed to sit down on the toilet before a rush of liquid left my body. I wasn't really sure if it was water or urine, to tell the truth. But after I realized that moving around on the seat made more liquid dribble out with no sensation of urinating, I guessed it had to be my water breaking.

I started to cry. A natural childbirth was so crucial to my dreams of our baby's arrival. I knew the hospital would wait only 24 hours after my water broke for my labor to begin on its own. After 24 hours, they would induce. I was worried that my labor wouldn't start soon enough.

Jerry had slept through the water breaking, but now my crying woke him up. We discussed things as calmly as I could and decided we would wait 12 hours for labor to begin naturally before contacting our obstetrician. Amniotic fluid continued to leak out, which I didn't expect. I found out later that your body continues to make more fluid, which of course will dribble out without a barrier in place.

We cuddled together in bed that morning and I dozed until about 7:30 a.m., when I felt it was a respectable hour to call our childbirth instructor for advice. I still didn't feel anything that might be called labor. But since my water had broken, I was worried about our decision to stay home. I was most concerned about cord prolapse, which can occur if the cord slips through the cervix, carried by the rush of amniotic fluid when the water breaks. If the cord becomes compressed, it can cut off the blood flow to the baby. After discussing my fears, our childbirth instructor suggested we listen for the baby's heartbeat with a stethoscope. Stethoscopes are readily available at medical supply stores and some drugstores, so we got into the car and drove to the closest one. Thirty minutes later, back at home, Jerry listened for the baby's heartbeat. At first he could only find mine, which of course only increased my anxiety. Then, at last, he found the other heartbeat. Our baby was all right! We could stay home.

As the morning progressed, we tried all of the old-wives'-tale tips for natural induction of labor: nipple stimulation, pressure on the roof of the mouth, pressure beside the Achilles' tendon, walking. We strolled up and down the street, talking about all the "what ifs."

Bradley teaches that the laboring woman should continue to eat if hungry and drink if thirsty. I had eaten breakfast and when we returned from our walk, it was lunchtime. But before preparing lunch, I felt like I needed to have a bowel movement. Once I was on the toilet, however, the sensation vanished.

After lunch, I asked Jerry to listen again for the baby's heartbeat and lay down on my back. Before he could find it, though, I got so uncomfortable, I had to get up. "Wait a minute," I thought. "What was that?" "That" was probably my second labor contraction, the first being the "urge" to have a bowel movement. It was 1:00 p.m.

By 1:30 in the afternoon I was hunched over on the toilet with Jerry pressing his fist as hard as he could into the small of my back, where it felt like someone was hitting me with a baseball bat. The counter-pressure of his fist eased the sensation. We had been in labor for less than 30 minutes, yet my contractions were only three minutes apart.

This was nothing like anything I had read or heard about. The first contraction had felt like a brief, light touch on the small of my back.

At 1:10, I picked up my copy of *What to Expect When You're Expecting* and started pacing circles around the house while re-reading the description of labor. Yes, it said labor could start with sensations in the back. (Somehow I had always imagined labor contractions were an abdominal thing.) By 1:20, I had already given up trying any of the labor positions advocated in my Bradley classes. The sensation that I had to have a bowel movement made anyplace other than sitting on the toilet seem impossible to me.

In retrospect, I was overwhelmed, yet still determined to achieve the natural childbirth of my dreams. So when Jerry timed the contractions and said they were already closer than the five-minute frequency we had agreed would be our cue to begin our 20-minute drive to the hospital, I told him, "I am not going to the hospital after only half an hour of labor!"

We tried the relaxation techniques we had learned in Bradley. We tried all the labor positions I had learned from *Active Birth*, by Janet Balaskas, a very helpful birthing book. Within minutes, however, my labor had progressed from vague sensations that had me wondering whether I could really be in labor to slamming contractions in the small of my back. The feeling was not of something building and releasing. It was either "there it is," with the force of being hit with a baseball bat or "now it's gone." Jerry will tell you I was not a quiet laborer. It felt better to make noise. Jerry said the noises I was making sounded like something from *The Exorcist*. I remember trying to breathe out and making a noise at the same time, a kind of breathing groan.

I spent the rest of my time at home on the toilet. When the contractions were a minute and a half apart and had been for half an hour,

Jerry decided to take control of the situation and insisted we go to the hospital. Between contractions, he loaded my things into the car. I hated to let him go and take away the pressure of his fist on my back, but I was glad he had made the decision to go to the hospital. It was around 2:30 p.m.

I can remember in vivid detail the red truck with a load of mulch that was driving slowly down the road ahead of us on the first stretch to the hospital. And I remember exactly how bad it felt to be sitting down during a contraction. My contractions did not slow down or stop during the drive, as I have heard sometimes happens.

At 3:00 p.m., when we arrived in the Labor and Delivery room at the medical center, the nurse gave me a hospital gown to put on and told me to relax during a contraction, which I assured her I was already trying to do. Jerry, my official "timer," tells me the contractions were about one and a half minutes apart from about 2:00 p.m. until the birth at 7:10 p.m. At this point, they all felt the same intensity to me.

I changed into the hospital gown in the bathroom, leaving my clothes in a heap (where I found them, untouched, hours later). Then the nurse asked me to lie back on the bed and she did an internal exam. (That was so very uncomfortable! There must be alternative positions that do not increase the mother's discomfort at this point.) The nurse told me she thought I was completely dilated, but she wanted a second opinion. I suppose because it was my first baby, she couldn't believe things were that far along. The second internal confirmed it: I was fully dilated, though the baby had not yet dropped into zero position, where the head is fully engaged within the pelvis. They told me to begin pushing. Jerry, remembering his training, asked me if I felt the urge to push. I said I really didn't know.

The nurse observed that the noises I was making, breathing groans, were actually suppressed pushing grunts. So I pushed, and it felt right. Pushing with the contraction did not hurt, but it did feel like work. I still could not sit or lie on my back without extreme discomfort.

At this medical center, they require an external baby heartbeat monitor to be in place for the duration of labor. The monitor is held in position by a belt stretched around the abdomen. Since the only pushing position I could comfortably use on the bed was a squat to keep me off my tailbone, the monitor kept slipping. The nurses told me I would either have to lie on my back or get an internal monitor installed. I didn't like either choice, but the lesser of the two evils was the internal monitor except that I had to lie on my back to let them attach it to the baby's scalp. Thankfully, that only took one or two contractions.

I developed a routine for dealing with the contractions. I would get up into a squat, push, and roll back to rest. Squat, push, rest. Squat, push, rest. Toward the end, I was depending upon Jerry to lift me into position. It was hard work. I drank from a sipper bottle of water I kept next to me. The room was full of people: our labor nurse, another nurse, two student nurses, and later, the doctor. One of the student nurses, a male, volunteered to help Jerry help me, and we both accepted his help gratefully. The student nurses, having yet to witness a natural childbirth in their internships, stayed past their normal quitting times to be there for our baby's arrival. Natural childbirths, unfortunately, are a rare commodity in this area.

I had absolutely no sense of modesty. The hospital gown was the usual flimsy affair that opened in the back, but I did not even worry if it was covering me in the front. I couldn't stand my hair falling into my eyes and wore a headband to keep it off my face, and a ponytail holder to keep it back. I wanted to see, so I was wearing my glasses. I was hot, but my feet were cold, so I kept my socks on. Jerry took one picture of me in labor, and I can assure you, I was not a pretty sight, though that didn't even cross my mind at the time.

After three hours of pushing and the baby's slow progress into the birth canal (checked periodically by internal exams for which the nurses insisted I had to lie back), the obstetrician from our practice came in. When he walked into the room and saw me pushing in a squatting position on the bed, he asked the nurses, "Where's the squatting bar?"

This was music to my ears. I had asked at the beginning for a squatting bar, having some memory of them from our hospital tour. The nurses asked, "What squatting bar?" I think the doctor actually went in search of it himself, and, shortly, they were breaking down the bed into a different configuration—a two-step affair—and had attached the bar. Now I was sitting on a ledge, kind of like sitting in a chair, and all I had to do to push with each contraction was to roll forward a little, put my weight on my feet, hold onto the bar, and push. That was heaven. And what a relief for Jerry, too, not having to pick me up each time into the squat.

This is my biggest complaint against the hospital. I think it was ridiculous that no one knew about the squatting bar. I also feel that the nurses could have provided more coaching about effective pushing techniques. Early in the process, I passed feces onto the disposable pad during a push, and grossed myself out. I wish the nurses had offered me an enema when I first arrived. From that point on, I don't think my pushes were as effective as they could have been. I was afraid of passing more feces, and I wasn't able to focus my pushes on the correct muscles.

The closest feeling I can compare to birthing a baby is having a very difficult bowel movement. I have heard the experts say it is not the same, but for me, it felt very close. The actual pushing felt much like straining for a bowel movement, and the passage of the baby down the birth canal felt like the pressure of something passing during a bowel movement. When the baby was crowning, it felt like I was holding something huge in my butt.

At 7:00 p.m., after four hours of pushing, the doctor told us he did not think my perineum was going to stretch enough to allow our baby to be born. We asked him to do a pressure episiotomy, that is an episiotomy without anesthesia. (I was already so numb, I didn't feel it.) After the cut, in the next contraction the baby's head emerged, face down, and then Jerry tells me the baby turned to look up at me. We had to wait a moment for the doctor to check on the position of the cord. Then, with one more contraction, the baby was born as I leaned back, sitting up on the bed.

I felt a sweet "zzzt-sting" piercing sensation as the baby slipped out. It was partly a feeling of release, partly the sting of salt in the episiotomy cut, partly the thrill of birthing. Since the doctor had asked me to lean back so he could see, I did not actually see the birth myself. I heard the doctor say, "It's a big boy!" It was 7:10 p.m. and we had been in labor for about six hours. We said, "Hello, Lucas Austin!"

Lucas was bloody and covered with vernix, the white cream that protects the baby's skin from exposure to the amniotic fluid in utero. The blood surprised me. I don't know if it was all from my episiotomy or not. The nurses wiped Lucas with a towel and put a little warming cap onto his head.

Within minutes, the doctor told Jerry it was time for him to cut the cord. Jerry was so proud to do that for Lucas. They lifted the baby up onto my abdomen, skin-to-skin, and covered us with a towel. The feeling of the warmth of his little body against mine is indescribable. Jerry and I sang, "Twinkle, Twinkle, Little Star," the song we had sung daily to him in the womb, and we swear Lucas smiled at us in recognition. Lucas rooted for my nipple and began suckling. What a joyful sensation.

The nurse told us Lucas's Apgar scores were 9 and 9 and that she never gave scores of 10, so his score was as close to perfect as could be.

While Lucas was still nursing, Dr. Miller told me to push again to deliver the placenta. I wasn't aware of feeling the placenta in the birth canal, but again, I felt a "zzzt-sting" sensation as it emerged.

Lucas watched my face as he nursed, and Jerry and I talked to him, telling him how much we had been looking forward to this moment. The doctor stitched up the episiotomy, which had torn just a little in addition to the doctor's cut. Once our baby was safely born, I was no longer worried about using drugs, so I let them give me a local anesthetic before stitching.

Once Lucas had finished nursing, Jerry snuggled with him. We had to stand our ground and remind the nurses more than once that our pediatrician had given his approval for us to keep our baby with us, as long as he was healthy, and he obviously was. Finally, after two hours, the nurses insisted it was time to weigh and measure him.

They had brought the scales into our room, so I saw the nurse place Lucas on them and heard her announce his weight: 9 pounds, 14 ounces. I was videotaping the action, and on the tape we hear my surprised "What?!" I had had no idea he was that big. He was 22 inches long.

Lucas roomed in with me for the entire hospital stay of 36 hours. I wanted to know when my baby woke up, so that I could offer him the breast and the comfort of my presence. We snuggled together in the hospital bed with the rail up. Sleeping that first night in the hospital was difficult due to the residual thrill of birthing (and my insatiable hunger!). I felt great, however.

The pure joy and satisfaction I felt for bringing my son safely and unharmed into the world stays with me to this day. I believe that staying drug-free enabled me to use my birthing muscles to their fullest extent, preventing unnecessary medical intervention. And it was a good start toward the close and warm relationship Lucas and I enjoy today.

BIRTH STORY
By Barbara Kozlowski, CNM

(I'm drowning)

And the midwife holds me in her arms and says

Yes it's hard isn't it you're doing so well

(And I'm surfacing)

And she says you're doing it exactly right

(And I'm drowning)

And she says you're taking such good care of your baby

(And I'm surfacing)

And she says yes this is how it is you'll live you're good and strong

(And I'm drowning)

And she says good good that's good

(And I'm surfacing)

And part of me says f_ _ _ you I'm dying here

(And I'm drowning)

And part of me says oh my god I AM doing this aren't I

(And I'm surfacing)

and part of me says LEAVE ME ALONE SAVE ME HELP ME

(And I'm drowning)

And part of me says this is the most incredible thing I've ever done

I can't believe I'm actually doing this yes yes YES

(And I'm surfacing)

And the baby comes in a long sea salt waterfall flood ocean
of sweat and tears and birth waters and blood

And I take her slippery warm wide-eyed amazed and knowing little
self against my EarthMother created-and-moved-the-
universe warm and billowy belly and tell her she's
wonderful and safe

And I follow her with a red and glorious afterbirth

And I think I DID IT! I AM TOTALLY INCREDIBLE! WE
WANT SOME PRIZES AND NEWS COVERAGE IN HERE!
DID YOU *SEE* THAT? WAS THAT *GREAT* OR WHAT?!

And the doctor writes

32-year-old grand II para I presents in active labor. Normal spontaneous
vaginal delivery of viable female LOA over intact perineum. Apgars 9 & 10.
Uneventful delivery.

Expectation vs. Reality

Don is a writer who lives in Massachusetts.
His wife, Cindy, is a professor of Spanish language and literature.
Their daughter was born in a hospital when Cindy and Don
were both 32 years old.

My daughter's birth was not exactly as I expected it to be. I had expected to cry when she was born, had perhaps even planned on it, which may have been the problem, because when the time came, I didn't cry. My wife and I had talked about keeping the placenta, using it to plant a tree, a Native American custom. That didn't happen either. Seeing it lying there on a tray after the birth, I would have believed the midwife if she had told me Cindy had just inexplicably ejected her liver—the thing was *huge*—but I couldn't quite bring myself to ask to have it wrapped up so I could take it home.

We left for the hospital just after midnight on a Monday morning. There was no traffic. It was late March, and I don't remember it being cold. The hospital was quiet, but the maternity ward was busy. Thinking back on it now, the hours between midnight and 6:00 were a bit surreal. We would find out later that while we counted contractions, two emergency C-sections had been performed, which explained the occasional screaming we'd heard. My wife was vomiting because of the pain, so at one point, she was given an antinausea injection. We passed the time in a private labor and delivery room, lights dimmed, trying to rest as much as we could, the midwife checking in and out periodically to monitor Cindy's progress, and giving us updates.

I WOULD LIKE TO SAY THAT I FELT IMPORTANT, EVEN ESSENTIAL. I FELT INSTEAD LIKE A PARTICULARLY INTERESTED THOUGH IMPOTENT BYSTANDER.

Despite a good intellectual knowledge of what's involved in childbirth, the books I had read, the hours spent in parenting preparation classes, I hadn't thought through what those hours in labor would be like for my wife. The pain I had anticipated; the messier aspects I knew about; what I hadn't thought about is how potentially embarrassing it could be to give birth, the degree to which a woman in labor is a spectacle open to virtually anyone working in the hospital who happens by. This isn't something my wife complained about, then or later, but I couldn't help being aware that, both physically and emotionally, Cindy spent most of her hours in labor quite intimately exposed. She had other things to think about, of course.

I think women are more owned by the experience of birth than men are. For me, there was the pull of a split imperative that I suspect other fathers share: I wanted to be as deeply involved in the experience as I could be, to even be emotionally taken over by it, and I wanted to stay calm enough and therefore sufficiently distanced to remain functional, to be helpful.

I did what I could—hunted up the midwife when Cindy needed her, periodically went and got additional ice chips, called friends and family at the appropriate moments. I would like to say that I felt important, even essential. I felt instead like a particularly interested though impotent bystander. I watched, I waited, I hoped.

Twelve and a half hours after we arrived at the hospital, as I held one of my wife's knees up near her ear, as I stroked the back of her neck, Rebecca was born. At 12:30 p.m., I cut the umbilical cord, a rubbery cable.

Holding her for the first time, moments after her birth, I wanted to see everything in her, this slick and squirming creature. Who was she? I was fascinated by her, enraptured, in love, in shock. I tried to take in what had just happened to me. I was a father now, and I felt as though I had gone immediately from being a child to being a parent, but somehow it was still a surprise, even after years of discussion and months of anticipation.

She was alert, moving her head around more than the rest of her body; her eyes flickered from sight to sight as she tried to take in where she was and what had just happened to her.

And, yes, she seemed intelligent, cognizant, beautiful, if still somewhat goopy, a whole new person sprung from us, a wealth of possibilities and potentials, untapped, but both perfectly clear and absolutely unimaginable. Look what we had done!

Five months after my daughter's birth, I wonder about what I mean to her—really mean to her; what she senses, believes, or feels about me, whether or not I have a fixed identity to her, or whether my value to her shifts with each task I perform. I just don't want her to need me physically, to feed and to clothe and to bathe her. I want her to need me emotionally, which is what I have wanted from the moment of her birth. How deeply etched is my face, my voice, my smell in her mind? A terrible burden to put on her perhaps. Or is it the most natural urge in the world?

Unbelievable Pain, Amazing Joy

*At the time of their first child's birth, Candace was 27
and David was 39. She had studied international relations
at Princeton, but was temporarily helping David and his
partners organize and computerize their painting and
renovating business. Their baby was born in a
hospital in Princeton, New Jersey
with a midwife's assistance.*

Having had Braxton Hicks contractions throughout the last four months of my pregnancy, I knew the contractions that began on the Wednesday night before I gave birth were different. They were not terribly painful, but they felt very strong and came every 10 minutes. However, I was able to sleep through them, and Thursday morning, David and I agreed that he'd go to work for a few hours to finish up some critical things, but that he would remain attached to his beeper. I called him at 11:00 a.m., ecstatic to say that the contractions were now about seven minutes apart, and that I'd be in touch. I went for a walk, hoping to encourage labor, but instead, the contractions stopped. By the time I returned home at 2:00 p.m., David was there waiting for me. I was very disappointed to tell him that we did not yet need to go to the hospital.

Thursday night at about 10:00, the contractions started again, much more intensely than the night before. These hurt! We tried to watch a movie between contractions, then went to bed. I slept a bit between the contractions, but was rudely awakened every 10 minutes or so by the pain. I did the deep breathing I had learned in my yoga pregnancy class, which helped, but at a certain point, I became a bit distraught and started crying. This woke up David, who hadn't been sleeping too well either. He said, "This looks like a good time to get into the bathtub." So at 2:00 a.m. I got into the tub and David started pouring water on my belly during the contractions. That helped a lot, and I stayed in the tub for at least three hours.

Our plan was for me to labor in the comfort of our home as long as possible so I could continue to eat, and could avoid medical interventions resulting from being committed to the hospital environment too early. So about 5:00 a.m. we took a dark morning walk around our neighborhood. It was painful to walk, but still bearable. Then I got back into the bathtub for a couple of hours while David continued to pour water over my belly. I thought I should eat something, but I didn't really feel like it. David made some toast and juice (which we ate) and packed some food and other things for the hospital, while I waited for some sort of discernible change.

By noon, my contractions were a consistent nine minutes apart (they had ranged from seven to ten minutes apart since the previous night) but they had not changed in intensity. They were very uncomfortable, even painful, but still bearable. I didn't think it was time yet to check into the hospital, but I wanted very much to be examined. I had to be reassured that I had progressed, at least a little. I wanted to know that I was 100 percent effaced, and dilated at least 1 or 2 centimeters. I felt that if I knew this, I could go on.

The midwife couldn't see me until 2:30 p.m., which seemed years away. When we arrived at the office, I had a much stronger contraction (probably brought on by the walk into the office). The staff, with whom I was now pretty friendly, made sympathetic comments. These words opened the floodgates for me and I cried out all my pain and anxiety and exhaustion. I felt like an overemotional woman, but the

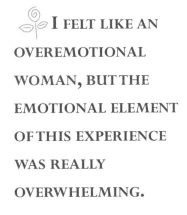 **I FELT LIKE AN OVEREMOTIONAL WOMAN, BUT THE EMOTIONAL ELEMENT OF THIS EXPERIENCE WAS REALLY OVERWHELMING.**

emotional element of this experience was really overwhelming. When Donna called me into her office, she did a cervical exam, and told me I was dilated between 3 and 4 centimeters. Yes! This was all worth it. I was going to have a baby!

About a minute later, I had the strongest, most painful contraction yet. A few minutes later, another. Several minutes more, another and another. These were incredible. I did not have control of my speech, my movements, or my thoughts during the pain. It felt as if my whole body resided in my stomach, which was now contracting. Powerfully. Painfully.

David was trying to encourage me to return home for a little while, but I didn't see how we could do that. Donna, upon seeing the pain I was in, suggested we go across the street to the hospital. It seemed that the cervical exam had brought on full labor. She said she'd meet us there in a few minutes.

Our walk through the underground tunnel was pretty uneventful, luckily. My contractions were bearable again, and I was really glad I didn't have to create a scene in front of innocent bystanders. I checked into the Labor and Delivery room, and the nurse did another monitor strip to make sure the baby was responding well to the contractions. Then she handed David a small pitcher he could use to pour water on my belly and directed us to the hospital bathtub. (The midwives had trained the hospital staff well!) The tub was disappointingly small, especially since I had read about birthing centers where mothers could undergo natural childbirth in deep, wide Jacuzzis. Worse, the temperature of the water was only tepid. No more relief from the nice warm water David had poured on me throughout the night. Maybe it would have been better to stay home longer I thought.

David went to get our things from the car, and Donna came in to pour the water on me. We chatted between my contractions, which were bad, but not too close together, six minutes apart, maybe. Then she left and David took over. I started getting frustrated and wanted to be checked again, so the nurse told me I would have to move to the bed, since Donna was also pregnant and couldn't bend over to check me in the bathtub. The walk to the bed was excruciating. I had the most violent contraction yet and couldn't stand on my own. Someone supported me and helped me get to the bed. When Donna returned, she expressed surprise that I had gotten out of the tub. That made me angry. Now I had lost my most comfortable place, and there was no way I could make it back there again. I wasn't going to go through *that* again. But I was at 7 centimeters. Maybe this was almost over.

By now the contractions were becoming absolutely unbearable. I lay on my side because that was the position I had taken when I got into the bed, and I did not dare move in any direction. I just took each contraction as it came and screamed and screamed. I had expected to use the slow yoga breathing throughout labor, but even when I was still at home, I found it was simply too painful to breathe deeply during a contraction. I could barely breathe normally. So I tried to breathe between contractions, but I completely gave up trying to

> **I JUST TOOK EACH CONTRACTION AS IT CAME AND SCREAMED AND SCREAMED.**

maintain any type of regular breathing during the pain. The only thing that felt good in my abdomen was to tighten and scream. You could euphemistically call this "using sound" (a technique covered in yoga class), but I think I was just screaming. By this point in my labor, there was hardly a break between screams, and no relief from the pain. This was worse than I imagined it would be.

Donna suggested I get back into the tub, but I couldn't imagine traveling such a long distance in this condition. I also knew that hospital regulations didn't allow the midwives to deliver babies in the bath, so I knew it was impractical as well. I don't think I even responded to Donna's suggestion. Feeling and hearing my pain, she asked me if I wanted something to help take the edge off. I had a gut feeling that if it hurt this much, it must be almost over. I also knew that the narcotics and analgesics given by injection do reach the baby's bloodstream, and that they don't help too much for the pain at this stage. "I don't know," I finally said, weakly. At least I didn't say yes.

Soon my screams were replaced by an animalistic deep grunting. This noise accompanied the pushing as beautifully as the screams had accompanied the earlier contractions. At 8:00 p.m., the nurse asked if I was fully dilated yet, and Donna answered that judging by the noises I was making, I was probably pushing already. She checked me again and I barely heard her say, "Just a rim left." Then I saw her hand move near me, and felt the warm liquid gush out, kind of a nice, messy feeling.

I know that David was there rubbing my head and touching my body to provide comfort, but I really was quite out of touch with reality. My consciousness had been altered by a combination of pain, the endorphins produced by my body to manage the pain, and oxytocin, the hormone that causes contractions. David's little massages didn't provide much relief, but I felt and appreciated his presence.

I continued to push with all my being, in sync with those unmistakable contractions that were screaming, "*Push!*" (Donna and the hospital nurse did not shout instructions at me as they do on *Emergency 911*.) Soon I could feel the baby's head against my perineum. It was exhausting to push, but I knew that pushing would end the pain. I mustered all my strength and pushed the head out with a loud scream. Donna pulled my hand down to feel the head covered with vernix, fluid, and lots of hair. At that moment I really didn't feel like exploring the baby—I just wanted it out, but now I can remember what the head felt like and can enjoy the feeling in retrospect.

Donna warned me that the hand was coming out with the shoulder. Another big painful push, and at 8:25 p.m. the rest of little Galit slid smoothly out, and she was placed almost immediately on my tummy.

I could hardly believe the pain was really over. And suddenly there was a breathing baby on my stomach. Feeling her weight, I knew she was real. Childbirth was over, and I put my arms around my beautiful new baby girl.

Whatever's Best for the Baby

*Diane was a 36-year-old graduate student at the time
of her first child's birth, a planned C-section performed in
a hospital in Carmel, New York. Her husband, Drew, 32,
was also a graduate student. Their baby was in the frank
breech position, and was also two weeks late. A cesarean
section takes only a few minutes to perform, but the
road to a planned one is much longer.*

My first pregnancy was perfect. Except for the first trimester, when I had morning sickness all day long, I glowed with more energy and well-being than I had in my pre-pregnant state. I worked out regularly with a pregnancy video, slept when I was tired, and ate a healthy diet.

I found my doctor through a friend who had recently been through her first pregnancy. He really loves delivering babies, and his enthusiasm inspired confidence. He also believes in using a natural approach whenever possible. His nurse told me that once, during a delivery, he screamed down the hospital hallway, "Where's the olive oil? I need more olive oil!" When the desk nurse asked if it was for his salad, he replied, "No! It's to rub the perineum, of course."

When I went for my 30-week checkup, I learned that my baby was presenting in the frank breech position (buttocks down). My first thought was, "What did I do wrong?" I had wanted to have the perfect pregnancy, and so far I had. Why did we have to be in the small percentage of breech births? We went home and read all the sections in my pregnancy books about C-sections that we had confidently skipped over before. The details of the surgery frightened me a little, but reading about the process helped us become familiar with it, so that if surgery became necessary, we wouldn't be going into it cold.

My friend Michelle, a Shiatsu massage therapist, recommended a special massage for my belly that she said might cause the baby to turn by itself. I also tried lying on the sofa with my feet up and my head down, as my doctor had recommended. But it was all for naught.

In my 38th week, the baby was still in breech position, and by now it was big, approximately 9 pounds, 2 ounces according to the sonogram. At my checkup, the doctor suggested we try an external cephalic version, where he tries to turn the baby manually. He explained the procedure and warned me that it would hurt, probably a great deal. But this 6-foot, over-200-pound man was confident he could do it. He told me he had successfully turned 11 out of 13 babies that year. He jumped up on the table, and it was only then that I realized he was going to use brute force to try to turn the baby. At the time I was hooked up to a sonogram machine, and the gentle rolling of the scanner over my jellied-up tummy was more my idea of a medical procedure.

Well, the good news is that the uterus is an amazingly strong muscle. The bad news is that when a 6-foot, 200-pound doctor is up on the table throwing his whole body weight into your uterus, you wish it wasn't quite so resistant to outside interference. My husband felt really helpless seeing me in obvious pain. After what seemed like forever, during which time I used all the Lamaze techniques we had learned about, bit through my lip, and raked my nails into my husband's hands, the doctor stopped because he was worried about stressing the baby too much. The baby had responded to this treatment by turning into the transverse position, which is straight across. The doctor was hopeful that given this head start, the baby would turn the rest of the way on its own. As I lay hooked up to the fetal monitor for the next few hours, I was really worried about my poor baby having been disturbed like that. A week later, when I was tilted back in a dentist's chair, the baby finally did turn, but back to the original butt-down position, with its head comfortably resting on my placenta. We were all disappointed, the doctor most of all, I think.

Well, it seems I can grow babies quite well, but they just don't want to come out. (My second baby was also late.) When we discussed our birth options at my 41-week appointment, the doctor and his colleague said they were willing to try a vaginal birth if I were really wedded to the idea, but in their opinion, given the position and size of the baby, its lateness, and the lack of any signs of labor, I would probably end up having a C-section anyway. When I asked what would be the safest way for the baby and they both answered, "C-section," I knew that's what I wanted to do. Our baby was fine, and I wanted to keep it that way. I was so relieved that this baby was finally coming out, and safely, that I welcomed the C-section. The only thing I worried about was the surgery itself, since I'd never had surgery before.

Once I agreed to the surgery, the doctors' immediate response was, "Okay, let's do it. Go get your pre-op blood work done, and we'll see you Monday morning at 6:00 a.m. in the hospital." I remembered the line, "Monday's child is full of grace—that's good for me!" It was kind of weird to know ahead of time the baby's birth date and its approximate weight. (I had undergone amniocentesis, but we had asked not to be told the sex.)

That weekend I felt both relief and apprehension. I had never been admitted to a hospital, and I did have some fear of the unknown, but underneath it all, I just kept joyfully humming to myself that in a very short time we would finally meet our baby.

I WAS SO ELATED AND APPREHENSIVE. AND I WAS READY TO GET THAT BABY OUT OF ME! THIS WAS THE BEGINNING OF MY 42ND WEEK.

We had pre-registered at the hospital, so on Monday morning, we were set up pretty quickly in my room. There was a scheduling snafu and the surgery was delayed until 1:00, but that was okay. I could not have tolerated being home anymore, I was so elated and apprehensive. I was so ready to get that baby out of me!

The nurses were great. One came into the room and reviewed with us what would happen before, during, and after the surgery. She explained the anesthesia, telling me that I would become completely numb below the waist, and that they would set up a screen before they made the incision so I wouldn't have to see it. My husband could be there if he wanted to (and he did). The nurse also assured us my doctors were excellent. Then the nurse who would monitor me during the surgery came in. She was wonderful. She was also a midwife, and was very interested in educating us about what was going to happen. The rest of our waiting time we spent walking up and down the hall, looking out the windows, talking. It was July and really hot and humid outside.

At 1:00 p.m., I walked into the operating room and sat down on the table. The room was tiny, cheerful, and crowded. It held Drew, my nurse, the anesthesiologist, his assistant, two doctors and their assisting nurses, the baby's doctor and his nurse and me—eleven people! The nurse told me to sit up and swing my legs over the side of the operating table, which was surprisingly narrow. She held my hands and helped me lean over and curve into the spiral position the doctor needed to ad-minister the spinal block. The effect of the drug was immediate. I felt a creeping numbness going down my legs. Minutes later, I lay down, with the needle still in place, which didn't bother me. The cloth screen was set up. Drew, wearing scrubs, sat to my left holding my hand, and soon everyone got to work. They offered to hold a mirror for me so I could watch the baby being born, but I declined.

The nurses described the procedure to me as it was occurring, step by step. The doctor made a small bikini incision just below my pubic hairline, which had been partially shaved. (My husband told me later that he was tempted to watch them make the incision, but found he ac-tually couldn't.) The doctor then put his hand inside to pull the baby out. My husband said he became frightened by how far the doctor reached inside me. Later, the doctor told us that Emma was really tangled up inside, which explains why he was making faces and grimacing, as if he were really struggling.

The baby was very high in my uterus, with her hands curled up under her. Nevertheless, in just a few minutes, Emma was born. All I felt was a slight tugging sensation and then the doctor was holding up this red, squalling, beautiful baby. Drew and I were crying and smiling—the rush of feelings was so intense. She had a perfectly round head, a bonus for not having to exit through the birth canal. We called her *bella facia de luna* ("pretty moon-face") because she was the only C-section baby that day, and thus the only bruise-free, lump-free, round-faced baby in the nursery. But she also had very long fingernails and toenails and was covered with meconium, all signs that the cesarean was warranted, even aside from her position. During a vaginal birth, she might have swallowed the meconium, resulting in a very serious infection, and the long fingernails suggested that she had become what is considered an "old" baby.

The pediatrician took her to the warming table for a quick examination, then the nurses wrapped her and gave her, all covered in goo, to Drew to hold. I was overjoyed to see her father holding her. Next, my placenta was removed and then I was being stitched back together. This took quite some time, but neither my husband nor I watched, nor can we remember how long it took. We were completely mesmerized by Emma.

As soon as the team was done stitching, I was propped up in bed and given my daughter to hold for the first time. I couldn't sit up on my own because of the incision in my abdominal muscles. I put her to my breast to nurse and she knew just what to do. Amazingly, so did I. So many of my friends had had trouble breastfeeding that I had been a little fearful I wouldn't be able to nurse well. What a joy that it was so easy.

Afterward, we were wheeled back to our room. The nurse came and took Emma to the nursery, with Drew and our brand-new video camera following. He captured Emma being weighed and measured and examined. She was 8 pounds, 14 ounces and 21 inches long.

We stayed in the hospital for three days. I was given an IV drip-on-demand for the pain, but I really didn't have much discomfort. It did take me several weeks before I felt completely recovered, though.

When I delivered my second baby vaginally, I was amazed at how I could immediately lift the baby unaided, and how soon afterward I could walk around. Not so after my cesarean. It was tough to temporarily lose the use of my abdominal muscles. But it was worth it!

A Pride Like No Other

*Catherine, 36 years old, and Mark, 37 years old,
a British couple, had their first child in London.
At the time, Mark was working for the British Broadcasting
Corporation. Catherine, a medical anthropologist who
studies birth practices in Nepal and throughout the world,
chose to have her baby in a hospital with the assistance
of her husband and a midwife. Mark shares his
recollections of the birth in the next story.*

Toward the end of my pregnancy I remember handing in my birth plan, walking out of the hospital to take the underground transport back home, and suddenly distilling all my preparation for labor into a simple sentence, which I found myself saying out loud: "A birth is like a marriage; you have to know what you want, but be prepared for anything."

Well, my baby was born on a Sunday, five days overdue, just when I had begun to think he would never arrive. The Friday before, I had

begun trying to move things along by a variety of means. An acupuncturist friend persuaded me that acupressure could easily help induce a birth,
so following her instructions, I tried self-acupressure on specific points of
my body. She also convinced me that it was time to stop working on my
research papers and to start focusing on the baby if I wanted him to come
out. (I was still writing research material for publication, cruising on a very
productive groove I had maintained throughout my pregnancy.) So I
shelved my papers, and tried to stimulate hormone production and uterine contractions by squeezing my nipples from time to time.

I had two contractions on Friday, but did not realize it at the time:
I was on the telephone both times and felt only a very bearable although unfamiliar ache.

Saturday night, my husband Mark and I went to dinner at my
mother's apartment, just around the corner, even though we were both
tired. Before we left, Mark had been playing the guitar and I had been
stretched out on the floor, listening to him. When we got to my
mother's, I went to the bathroom and found I had lost my mucous plug,
although once again I did not realize what was happening to me at the
time. I called out to my mother and Mark, and then burst into tears because the mucus was dark brown, not at all the color I had expected. I
thought this was perhaps meconium, a sign that things were going
wrong. We phoned a midwife friend of ours, and she reassured me that
the color was normal. So we proceeded with dinner, although I had
little appetite. When we returned home and prepared for bed, it seemed
that my contractions had started. They were about five minutes apart
and affected an apparently large muscle area. They were painless, and I

was puzzled, not really knowing what to expect; could mild, but frequent, contractions be the real thing?

We started noting down the times of the contractions, and yes, they were five minutes apart, each lasting about 20 seconds. I asked Mark to hook me up to the TENS machine we had rented. This machine was supposed to cut down pain by means of an electrical current across the spine. It was battery operated and portable. He fitted the four electrodes to my back and we went to bed. As I got up again to write down my contraction times, my waters broke—plop—running all down my leg and onto the carpet. It was so sudden I don't think I can ever forget it! I rushed to the bathroom, and called Mark to come help me figure out what to do next. We decided to call the

THE FIRST CONTRACTIONS WERE PAINLESS, AND I WAS PUZZLED, NOT REALLY KNOWING WHAT TO EXPECT; COULD MILD, BUT FREQUENT, CONTRACTIONS BE THE REAL THING?

hospital and to go there immediately, as my contractions, now four minutes apart, seemed frequent, anyway frequent enough for us. I called my parents and told them I would call them again from the hospital. I was still not convinced this was actual labor, but wanted to take all the right steps. I felt no actual pain, just trepidation.

For maternity patients who have no car, the hospital offers ambulance service. So we called an ambulance to come pick us up and went downstairs to wait. There I was, standing on Fore Street in the middle of the night, in the middle of the city, leaning against a concrete wall with my little red bag at my feet. My contractions were frequent but still quite bearable. We whizzed to the hospital in the ambulance, arriving at what must have been about 11:00 p.m.

We were admitted to the labor ward, where I was examined. A midwife told me that I was 1 centimeter dilated. Now the contractions started getting severe. This was no picnic. But the midwives, none of whom I recognized, were very efficient. I walked over to my birth room (I was pleased not to be offered a wheelchair!) and found it was more spacious and less daunting than the one I had visited during my prenatal classes. I had no wish to request a birth pool, a large tub where I could relax during contractions. That would have meant disconnecting myself from the TENS machine, which I did not want to do. I felt strong. This was it! I was stepping into the unknown.

When a doctor examined me a few hours later, I had dilated to 6 centimeters. It was difficult to tell exactly how much time had passed; there was a clock on the wall, but I was too focused on what was happening in my body to pay much attention to it. However, by now I had gotten the hang of my contractions. As each one started, I would count breaths: the first three were bearable, even easy, breaths four to ten were painful, and from ten onward they were *very* painful. I knew I had to get to breath number 17, and then the contraction would wane. I was told I was having double contractions, one right after the other. Mark was helping by holding me, his hand very tight on my back, and saying to me, "I've got you . . . I've got you . . ." over and over again.

Trouble started when the midwives hooked me to a monitor and found that the baby's heart rate was dipping, sometimes quite low, during my contractions. It could be that the hospital monitor did not pick up the fetal heart rate properly when I moved or when the baby moved. Unlike my modern, portable TENS machine, the monitor kept me confined to the bed and fit poorly, with straps and belts. It looked like it came from a field hospital in the 1940s. I was told to lie on my back and stay still (not at all what I wished for or had envisaged). Two doctors now tried to stick an electrode onto the baby's head in utero so they could more accurately monitor the fetal heart rate. But they gave up on the idea, saying, "Can't do anything, he's moving so much in there."

Then they told me they wanted to break my waters. That confused me, since I thought my waters had already broken; was there another layer or sac? I could have asked for an explanation, but I didn't bother: my mind was tracking more important things. In any case, they were not able to do so. Each time they approached either me or the baby inside me, his heart rate would jump to a normal steady rate. And each time they left the room, the heart rate would dip and look erratic, until the midwife on duty decided to buzz the doctors again. Of course, each time the doctors came into the room, I was asked to lie still on my back, and every time they left, I would turn back over onto my knees. I was happier with my back turned to the rest of the room. All my clothes were torn off by now, and I was holding the headrest of the bed and feeling the pressure of my husband's hand on my back, coping with contractions and glancing from time to time at the monitor to see how far the fetal heart rate was dipping. At one point the doctors came in and took a blood sample from a nick made to the baby's head and got a reading of his oxygen levels from the fetal blood. The levels were normal. They left the room, came back when the midwife buzzed them again, and took a second fetal blood sample, which was also normal. Then they left, giving up on the need for intervention altogether.

But in the meantime they had tempted me with an epidural. They had played the "good cop, bad cop" routine, the male Nigerian doctor acting the supportive and concerned part, the male Caucasian being more forceful. I ignored them for a while, to the point of rudeness. My back was turned to them, and I did feel that conversation was beyond me at this point. Eventually, between contractions, I managed to ask them, "Doesn't an epidural place me at greater risk of an intervention?" The reply was a solemn, "Madam, you already are at great risk of an intervention." I glanced at the monitor and its flashing heart rate values. But I told them I preferred to wait awhile and to think about it.

After they left, I kept wanting to ask for the epidural when I got to the painful number 17 breath of the contraction, but then I would recover at breath number 22, feel better, and think I could handle one more contraction. Each time I waited for the contraction to subside and told myself I could last for just one more. Psychologically it was like swimming lengths in an Olympic-size pool: when your body is exhausted, you tell yourself you will swim just one more length, but then you turn around and swim yet another, and then another until you have completed the target number of laps.

But what was my target in labor? How many hours? Because the ward supervisor had taken a break from duty and had been replaced by another midwife, I told myself I'd wait until her return, scheduled at 3:00 a.m., before asking for an epidural. She came, but she was half-an-hour late, and when she examined me, she told me, "You're near the end. The baby is going to come out now."

I truly realized I was getting toward the end of labor when she told my husband to turn off the fan, so the room could warm up for the baby. I never asked for that epidural. All I had for pain relief was the TENS machine (at one point I nearly electrocuted myself as I accidentally jumped the voltage up).

After seven hours in the hospital, the second stage of labor was just 26 minutes. First, I suddenly felt I was going to vomit, then I felt a pressing bowel movement, and I cried out to the midwife for help. She told me it was the baby coming, but I thought not, and indeed I passed feces into the pan she brought me. I was still on the bed, hooked to the damn monitor. Then I felt what felt like a *huge* bowel movement, and I knew that that was the baby coming. I felt a little hysterical, because this was something else, a sensation that was new and unexpected. The midwife was telling me to push hard and not to pant or try to avoid a tear, because she feared that the umbilical cord was around the baby's neck, which would explain why his heart rate had been dipping. So I pushed, a mighty four times and, suddenly, felt real physical exhaustion.

At that moment I thought that perhaps the birth was never going to happen, the baby was never going to come out. I remember collecting myself, deciding to push really hard next time, and to give it all I had. I called to the midwife, "Come on, let's get on with it now!" and my husband told me afterward how surprised he was at my resolute tone. Then abruptly, I felt something dissolve and fizzle out inside me. I cried out in fear to the midwife, "What are you doing?!" But it was the baby's head coming through, and the body slipping out, and there he was, our newborn. The cord was not around his neck. For some reason, the first thing I did was to look at the clock on the wall and note the time of his birth: 6:14 a.m.

I turned around to lie on my back. Mark cut the cord with some big scissors in two snips. The baby was free and was taken to the back of the room to be bathed and weighed and given his Apgar tests. Because I had taken oxytocin tablets to precipitate the release of the placenta, I now started shaking uncontrollably and my teeth were chattering. I remembered that the midwives had asked me to sign a consent form sometime during labor: it had felt bizarre, putting my signature to a piece of paper in the middle of having contractions, stark naked, showing my posterior for everyone to see. Although I had been told much about the current research on oxytocin tablets, I did not know that I would have to sign a consent form in the middle of labor. In any case, the placenta came out, and I asked to see it: it looked like a huge blue and red fleshy abalone. It was enormous.

ABSURDLY, I FELT QUITE PROUD OF MY TEAR, AS IF IT WERE A WOUND FROM SOME GREAT AND GLORIOUS BATTLE.

I can't remember much after that, but I think they gave me the baby and that he breastfed. They also sewed me up—three stitches for a

second-degree tear. The sheets were all bloody, but I didn't care: I had
come through and so had the baby. Absurdly, I felt quite proud of my tear,
as if it were a wound from some great and glorious battle. I got up to have
a bath, staining the floor, but feeling wonderful, leaving Mark to hold our
bundle of baby. Then we phoned home to spread the good news.

I was ready to move from the delivery ward to the recovery room. I
picked up my bags, but the midwife told me not to carry them. In something of a daze, I replied that since Mark was holding the baby, I had to
carry the bags, but she firmly insisted that I carry the baby and let Mark
carry the bags. So I took the baby from Mark and off we went, passing
the doctors on the way. They congratulated me and asked if the baby
had a name. No, he didn't, yet. With a smile, the Nigerian doctor said
I should name him "Trouble."

I walked out of the labor ward, a woman in control, feeling a tremendous sense of achievement. It felt like I had been dropped onto a train
that was hurtling 400 miles an hour in dark tunnels, where it was imperative that I keep a cool head, get to the driver's seat, and steer a course as
best I could. There was no way I could say, "Just a minute, I don't want to
be here. I want to get off this train and take a later one." It had been a
matter of life and death that I stay in control. And I had done it.

That night, I paced the corridors up and down with my baby, too
much in awe of him to think of getting any sleep, too elated at having
avoided medical intervention, like my mother and grandmother and
the Nepali women I knew from my work. I felt extraordinarily blessed
and lucky. This baby had invited himself into our family, after ten years
of marriage. All my labor pains were already forgotten: I wanted to birth

him all over again, it had gone by so quickly, and it had been so wonderful. I wanted to play back the moment when the baby left my body,
to understand what had been happening, to savor the moment. I felt a
tremendous sense of achievement, of absolute accomplishment. I had
given birth to a child, and I felt extraordinarily proud.

Changed Forever

At the time Dominic was born, Mark was doing media research for the BBC World Service. For five years, Catherine and Mark had a commuter marriage, traveling to be together on weekends because their jobs were in different cities. But after their son was born in a London hospital, they were inspired to create a permanent home for their family. Mark left his position with the BBC, and he and Catherine bought a house near her university. Mark eventually returned to school to study music.

I remember seeing Catherine's face flushed with the strain of it, beads of sweat breaking out on her forehead, and thinking how tough she was. I remember the midwife, Sue, a small, burly Asian woman, and thinking what an incredibly tough job it must be to deliver babies for a living. I remember all the bits of technology lying around the delivery room, the shiny tools and tubes we didn't use, the boxes of swabs and tissues we did, the little machine recording Dominic's heartbeat like a seismograph, the doctors and nurses who came in and out of the room, scrutinizing the data, trying to figure out what was going on inside my wife. I remember all the stories we'd heard and read about childbirth, ranging from a woman who had died in a London hospital like the one we were in to another who had gone through a birth successfully all by herself under a tree in the middle of the Kalahari Desert, worrying about the possibility of being attacked by hyenas. But what I tend to go back to most strongly now are the moments and places that took on meanings I didn't anticipate they would have had, or which fundamentally changed the way I regard my wife and myself.

For instance, I remember the place we waited for the ambulance to come and take us to the hospital. To anyone else, it is just another dull piece of urban fabric. But to us, it has turned into a place of significance. It is a curbside entrance to a subterranean parking lot in the middle of the city of London. There's ordinary pavement next to an ordinary street, a row of street lights facing a row of parking meters, a waist-high concrete wall enclosing a row of bushes and a soot-stained tree. That night one side of the street was a wall of neon-lit office windows and the other a block of dark apartments. A few cars whooshed by. Some drunken voices sang a soccer song in the distance, accompanied by a police siren. Catherine leaned against the wall and I put my hand on the base of her spine and pushed to ease the pain of the contractions. I remember us laughing at one point. I made a joke about the situation we were in, standing in the middle of a big city, giving birth on the pavement while people passed by on their way to the cinema. Now whenever we go by that place, we remember the night we waited for the ambulance there. Sometimes we even stop there for a moment, with the city roaring around us, and call up the memory. It's become the place we left from and returned to after the birth, and in a symbolic way, it's the place where we began to turn a corner in our lives together.

I also vividly remember my first sight of my son. I saw the top of his skull, an oval-shaped patch of gray skin, wet and matted with black hair. The midwife and I were looking at the top of his head as it first appeared between Catherine's thighs. I remember thinking how strange the situation was, staring at Catherine's backside with someone I'd only known for eight hours. But by this time, we'd achieved that rare form of intimacy shared by two people who have cleaned up excrement together at three in the morning. By this time, Catherine was naked, on all fours, with her elbows up on the back of the bed frame. She was yelling things like, "Okay, Sue, let's go," before a contraction started. I kept kneading the base of her spine, mopping her forehead. I remember telling her, "I can see his head! I can see his head!" A short time later, she yelled frantically, "What's happening? What's happening?" and I said, "He's coming out," and then he slipped out fast, all dripping and crying. Sue picked him up and we helped Catherine turn over and she put him on Catherine's belly.

I remember Sue asking me if I wanted to cut his umbilical cord. I took the tool she handed me and asked her if he'd feel it, if there would be any pain for him, and she said no. The scissors were razor sharp, shaped like a crescent, and I tried them out a few times before I did it. The umbilical cord was clamped, and he was breathing and sobbing a little. Catherine was looking at him for the first time and he was still a part of her. I cut the cord between them. Then I remember holding him while Sue sewed up some tears in Catherine's vaginal tissue.

Shortly after, Catherine had a cup of tea and then she walked out of the delivery room slowly, carrying our son up to her bed in the maternity ward. It was a dignified way to end her performance, a bit like a football player standing up and walking back into the game after sustaining a bad injury. I felt and still feel impressed by it.

SHE WALKED OUT OF THE DELIVERY ROOM SLOWLY, CARRYING OUR SON. IT WAS A DIGNIFIED WAY TO END HER PERFORMANCE. I FELT AND STILL FEEL IMPRESSED BY IT.

I remember going home for a shower and a rest after she and the baby were settled into bed. I walked out of the hospital at around 8:00 on a Sunday morning. There was hardly any traffic. I started walking in the direction of our flat, hoping to find a taxi. It was a crisp, clear morning and I had been up all night. I eventually hailed a cab and the driver asked me where I wanted to go. "Where to, guv?" I got in and as we pulled away, something broke in me. I felt this great joy rise up in my heart, but at the same time, I was totally exhausted. I sat in the back of the taxi in tears, looking out at London, shattered and astonished, thinking about what we'd just done, bringing another person into being. I remember realizing that the left side of my body was sore, seized up from pressing on Catherine's lower spine for ten hours. I remember thinking how special the day was for me, and how ordinary it probably was for the man driving me home.

Nine months into his life I can recall thinking of Dominic as a piece of Catherine's biology, something that had to come out of her, something I wanted to help launch into life. We saw him in scans, on TV screens in hospitals, and we felt his kicks in the womb. We went to childbirth preparation classes and practiced various birth positions to help him get out. We worked with Sue and several other people monitoring his birth, looking at each other, talking about it, easing our son into the atmosphere. I don't remember being nervous or worried. I knew that one way or another we were going to get through it, like any of the other challenges we'd faced together over the past decade. So I just took care of my wife as best I could and tried to provide her with some strength and encouragement when she needed it.

Now our son is here with us, and I feel he is also somebody I want to help. He's no longer the wrinkled red baby Sue handed me in the delivery room. Now he laughs and wails and bangs his fists on the table. He lays his head down on my chest and falls asleep. We're out on the street corners together and I'm holding him against my stomach, remembering his birth while the traffic swirls by.

A Surprise Home Birth (1954)

*Carolyn was a 25-year-old homemaker in 1954
when her first baby was delivered by her mother
at her parents' home in Queens, New York, two weeks early.
Carolyn's husband, a 24-year-old carpenter,
was at work in Connecticut when the baby came.
Interestingly, Carolyn had also been delivered at home
by her grandmother 25 years earlier.*

When I was pregnant, we expectant mothers had only a small paperback Dr. Spock book for reference. His pregnancy guidelines were too vague to be very useful. I don't remember ever reading a complete outline of the human birthing experience. I never knew there were special breathing exercises to help with labor. The idea that your husband could participate in the birth, or that he could even be in the same room with you, was unheard of in the early fifties.

My husband and I had built a lovely two-bedroom home in Connecticut. Since moving there, we would travel two and a half hours, twice a month, to visit my parents in Queens, New York. My mother's birthday is August 25, so I had scheduled our visit for that weekend. My baby wasn't due until September 15, so we didn't expect anything unusual to happen.

I was uncomfortable on the trip down on Saturday. It seemed like the baby couldn't settle down. I had some cramps and felt a lot of activity going on inside me that I did not understand.

Saturday night I wasn't able to find a comfortable position for sleeping. The cramps had continued on and off. Sunday evening, I did not feel better, so I suggested to my husband that he return to Connecticut to work and leave me with my mother to rest for the week. He could return Friday after work and we would be able to drive home Saturday morning in time to keep my Saturday afternoon doctor's appointment. He agreed that

THE IDEA THAT YOUR HUSBAND COULD PARTICIPATE IN THE BIRTH, OR THAT HE COULD EVEN BE IN THE SAME ROOM WITH YOU WAS UNHEARD OF IN THE EARLY FIFTIES.

sounded like a good idea and he left me with my parents in Queens. I spent a leisurely week there, experiencing occasional cramps.

Friday, September 3, was a beautiful, clear, sunny day: good walking weather. Over our morning coffee, my mother and I decided to go shopping. My parents' home was situated on a hill, and the walk down to the main street was invigorating. I remember mentioning to my father before he left for work at 6:00 in the morning that I had experienced a number of back pains during the night. The walk downhill really relieved my back.

Mom and I stopped at a local cafe to have lunch. I am a Catholic, and we still observed Friday as a meatless day back then, so I ate a tuna salad sandwich.

We did a little more shopping before we tackled the walk home. By the time we arrived at the top of this relatively small hill, I was huffing and puffing. After putting our purchases away, I suddenly felt lightheaded. I knew I was tired and now I felt queasy, too, but I blamed the mayonnaise in my sandwich for my discomfort. After all, I wasn't due for two more weeks. I decided to lie down for a while; it was about 3:00 p.m.

Mom figured this was a chance for her to phone her sister, Nell, for a chat. Outside the bedroom door was a small square foyer with a phone bench. From the bed, I could see Mom standing in front of the bench, dialing Aunt Nell's number, with her back to me. She did not see me trying to get up off the bed. It seemed the refill of iced tea I had had at lunch had been too much—I had to get to the bathroom—fast! I felt like my bladder was going to burst. I rolled to the edge of the bed, put my legs over the side and attempted to stand up. A sharp, knifelike pain in my lower abdominal area suddenly doubled me over, face down, on the bed, where I waited for it to pass.

My mother has difficulty hearing, and she had her good ear to the phone and her back turned toward me, so she could neither see nor hear my plight, so I picked up my slipper and threw it at the wall beside her. At that moment, my water broke. I saw the puddle on the floor. I slipped

126

to my knees. Mom turned around and, startled by the sight she saw, slammed the phone down without a word of explanation to her sister.

Then things began to happen fast. Mom scurried around looking for some newspaper to place under me. I still could not get onto the bed—and did not try to. Mom started muttering to herself. I asked her what she was saying. She told me her mother had delivered me at home, so she was running over in her mind what Grandma had done. She was saying, "Got to tie the cord. Need clean scissors. Need a piece of cotton for tying. First, I need alcohol for sterilizing."

While she was hunting for what she needed, she was also trying to get through to her doctor, but she kept getting a busy signal. When I was having a contraction, she would run back to be with me for it. She kept me talking, trying to distract me from my pain. Once, she gave me some warm tea to make me feel better. Sipping slowly was soothing.

Then she would go back to remembering what Grandma had done for her when I was born. Grandpa had to put scratch marks on the bedroom door to prove to the younger children when they returned from school that the stork had been there to deliver the baby. We laughed about that and said that was one European custom we didn't need to follow anymore.

Although I was in labor for about two hours, it didn't seem that long. There was pain and rest, pain and rest. I did not consider it pain when I was going through it. I was inexperienced and also enormously awed by what was happening.

We never timed the contractions. I just rolled with the punches. I knew they kept getting closer in the last hour, until I could hardly catch my breath toward the end. I remember my mother on the floor holding a flashlight. When she could see the baby's head, she told me to push.

I delivered my baby, on my knees. It was a girl. Mom made a good catch. Then she gasped, because this messy little thing was all blue and white. She unwrapped the cord and quickly turned the baby upside down. She gave her a slap, and then I heard my baby's lovely first cry.

Aunt Nell had been phoning throughout this time until Mom finally had a free moment to answer the phone. She was excited by the news and said she'd be on her way over shortly.

Mom had taken the white cotton tie strips from the inside of her housecoat to use for tying the cord, sterilized them by putting them in a cup of alcohol. After tying the cord and giving me my baby girl, Mom again tried her doctor's number. This time she got through. She quickly asked for her doctor and was informed that he was on vacation. All that had happened up to this point finally hit her, and she began to sob into the phone. The nurse assured her that the doctor's substitute was a very capable young man who had studied under her doctor. He got on the phone immediately and started asking questions. Then he said he'd be over in 10 minutes. We were so busy trying to clean my new baby, it seemed like no time at all before he arrived.

The doctor examined my little girl thoroughly. He gave Mom an A+ and a hug for a beautiful delivery. There was no need for anyone to go to the hospital. We phoned my best friend and asked her to bring us some supplies from the drugstore.

We had not been able to reach my husband. He was already en route to the city. When he arrived at about 6:30 p.m., we had a surprise for him.

Two for One

Nan, a 32-year-old American woman
married to Soren, a Danish man, delivered twins vaginally
in a hospital in Denmark. At the time she was between careers
as a financial consultant and a translator/writer.
Her husband is a dairy engineer.
She writes, "I included a description of the week on
the maternity ward to show just how long it can take to
bond with your newborns. I think first-time mothers need
to know that bonding may not be automatic."

I found out I was carrying twins during a routine sonogram examination in my 17th week. Luckily, I had the perfect conditions for carrying twins: I wasn't working at the time and we had no other children yet.

My pregnancy went well. My desire for just about everything unhealthy disappeared. Instead of drinking tea I drank milk, I took vitamins, and I napped every single day. I rode my bike for both exercise and transportation.

Just as the 38th week began, my water broke. It was midnight. I remember thinking I heard (but it was probably more that I felt) a little pop, just like a balloon quietly bursting, and suddenly I thought I had to pee. When I reached the bathroom, there was water running down my legs, but even though my bladder had gotten weaker, I was quite sure I wasn't urinating. After sitting on the toilet for a few minutes, I went back into the bedroom and told my husband, Soren, that I thought my water had broken. He didn't really believe me and went into the bathroom to look for himself. Then he was convinced, so he called the hospital to find out what we should do next.

I was lying in bed shaking violently, and when the midwife asked to speak to me on the phone, I could barely answer her. I asked her if I was supposed to shake like that, and she said I was probably just nervous. I could actually hear my teeth rattling against each other. In spite of the weekly examinations I had received throughout the previous two months, no one had ever told me whether or not baby A's head was engaged, that is, whether it had descended into a secure position within the pelvis. Because we didn't know if this had occurred, I was instructed to come into the hospital right away. They told us to call an ambulance, but we decided that was a little too dramatic. We hadn't prepared a bag, so we spent about 20 minutes packing, then drove to the hospital with me reclining in the front seat. The drive took about 20 minutes and the first contractions started about halfway there.

I had been having Braxton Hicks contractions for quite a while before that night. I didn't even know I was having them until, during one of my examinations, a monitor picked up the two babies' heartbeats plus my uterine contractions. After that, I learned to recognize them, but they didn't hurt. During the final three weeks before the birth, however,

I did get painful contractions after having an orgasm. They kept me up all night each time. The contractions I had in the car were different, like menstrual cramps. I noticed them, but they weren't really painful.

We arrived at the hospital at about 1:00 a.m. A midwife and a midwife trainee greeted us on the maternity ward. They wanted to put us in the biggest birthing room (which looked very technical and unfriendly), since twin births usually end up having a lot of onlookers. But I asked for, and was allowed to use, one of the other rooms, which are furnished more like bedrooms, with attractive wallpaper, ordinary furniture, a bathtub, a radio/tapeplayer, and potted plants. I told them I was afraid of using anesthesia and said that of course I'd have to live with full anesthesia if a cesarean became necessary, but that I wasn't interested in any drugs that might make me woozy. They examined me and found that I was 3 centimeters dilated. The midwife said, "This one will go quickly." They put a monitor on me to check the babies' heartbeats, and we were left alone to wait.

We did crossword puzzles, we played backgammon; we were bored and impatient, and the contractions were getting more and more like bad menstrual cramps. I dutifully used my breathing exercises. I tried getting into the bathtub, but lying still didn't seem to help, so I got up again pretty quickly. Three hours later, they examined me again. Unfortunately, I had not dilated any further. I was still determined to let things follow their natural course, so I said no thanks to an offer of oxytocin, a hormone that causes the uterus to contract.

By 5:00 a.m., we were getting tired, my contractions were getting stronger, and the midwives were changing shifts. We were introduced to a new pair of midwives, an older lady who seemed very tough and a younger trainee. They offered me sterile water injections in my back for the pain. In retrospect, I hadn't yet found out what real pain was, but at the time I thought my pain was bad enough to warrant some relief. They said the injection would feel like a bee sting, and that after I had gotten one, I would also have to get the other: was I still sure I wanted it? Unfortunately, I said yes.

I absolutely do not recommend these injections. (I don't think they are used in the United States.) The needles hurt like hell going in (Soren says I screamed like a pig), much more than the pain they were supposed to relieve. They were very effective for about three hours, but then their effect wore off. That may have been the most painful part of the whole experience. After the third hour, when they asked me if I wanted more, my response was, "Are you crazy?" I was checked again to see if I had dilated any more. "I'm almost afraid to say it," said the midwife. Still only 3 centimeters.

I had talked to a number of people about their birth experiences while I was pregnant, and people had widely different experiences to relate. But there was one thing that really struck me: the worst experiences were related by women for whom the process had dragged on so long that they became exhausted. The ones who didn't think it was that bad were women who had relatively quick labors. It seemed to me that the outcome was related less to the pain suffered or the medical procedures than to the labor's length and to the level of exhaustion.

With this in mind, I decided that since we were already so tired, it would be a good idea to let them give me some oxytocin. They said that

I would have to have it later anyway, because they always use it to get baby B out as quickly as possible. Therefore I would have an IV no matter what. They also wanted me to have the heart monitor on the babies again for 20 minutes.

After listening to two identical heartbeats for quite a while, they finally realized that they were listening to baby B's heart twice. Baby A was so far down in the birth canal that they couldn't monitor his heart from the outside, so now, in addition to the IV needle in my hand and the two monitors on my stomach (one for baby B and one for my contractions), they also placed a wire up into my vagina and attached it to baby A's head to monitor his heart. (It fell out about five times, and he had scabs on his head for a few weeks afterward.) It must have looked pretty comical every time I had to pee, because I had to roll the machine and IV bottle to the toilet along with me.

My contractions were pretty painful at that point and I began to hyperventilate, so my memories are somewhat jumbled. My husband watched the monitor and told me when a contraction was starting. He could also tell me when it was peaking, which helped me a lot, since I knew the pain would recede after that. I don't know why I hyperventilated, but spots appeared before my eyes and my hands and legs became numb. I got really scared; I was afraid I would pass out. They told me I wouldn't pass out, and I didn't, but they wanted me to breathe into a bag. I had a little trouble doing that with everything else that was going on.

Time was going very slowly. I was getting very tired and I was having trouble dealing with the pain. The pain would just swoop over the middle of my body, and it would take all my strength to get through the contraction. Then it would go away again and everything would be fine. I still had some time between contractions, so I was able to relax a little, but they were getting closer and closer together. I have to admit that because I was able to keep speaking Danish throughout the whole thing, I did not feel that bad. Otherwise, I would have switched to English. But I did scream a lot. Soren said he was afraid that the other women arriving after me would turn around and go home when they heard me. For me, it was like being on a roller coaster: it makes you feel better to scream. Screaming was a choice, not a sign of total desperation.

At some point, someone suggested that I try laughing gas. I was against the idea, since I had tried it once at the dentist's and hated it. I also thought I would get all weird and high, and I already felt a bit that way from hyperventilating. But finally I agreed to try it, and all I can say is that I became very friendly with that mask! I discovered that if I inhaled very deeply just before the peak of the contraction, it took the pain away completely. That worked great up until the very end, when the contractions were coming so quickly that I couldn't take deep breaths.

It was hard for Soren to see me in so much pain and to be so helpless. Around 11:30 a.m., the midwives suggested that he take a break and I said it was okay. He got a cup of coffee and relaxed a bit. After he came back, I started having the urge to push, and I don't think the midwives were terribly helpful because they hadn't given me any idea of how far we had gotten or how much more I would have to endure before I'd be allowed to push. When you're in pain like that, that kind of information is crucial. The last time they had told me anything I was only 7 centimeters dilated.

Apparently, the pressure of two babies and two placentas had brought on the urge to push before I was completely dilated. It was very difficult to have the urge and not be allowed to push, while having rapid and painful contractions. The only comforting thing I can say in retrospect is that when you get to that point, it's almost over. A few times, I told them that I would only endure one more contraction and then I was stopping. I think they had heard that kind of talk before.

At about 12:30 p.m., about 12 hours into my labor, I moaned once again, "Why can't I push?" and finally the midwife said, "Okay, push!" It was a big relief to be able to start pushing with my contractions. For me, it felt a lot like I had to have a bowel movement really badly, but it wasn't painful.

I think it was about at this point that they called in "the crew": the chief obstetrician, a pediatrician, a nurse, and a nurse's aide. We saw the anesthesiologists a few times, but they stayed discreetly outside the door, waiting to hear if an emergency cesarean would become necessary. They set up their equipment, but that didn't really bother me.

> **A FEW TIMES, I TOLD THEM THAT I WOULD ENDURE ONLY ONE MORE CONTRACTION AND THEN I WAS STOPPING. I THINK THEY HAD HEARD THAT KIND OF TALK BEFORE.**

What did bother me was having all those people watching. Everyone had told me that I wouldn't care at all by that time, but I did. They had given me an enema when I arrived (it was optional), so my bowels were empty, but I was still convinced that I was doing it all wrong and that I would have a bowel movement on this table with all these people watching.

Since they wanted to continue monitoring the babies' heartbeats, I ended up giving birth lying on my back, which was definitely not what I had planned. Each time I had to push, Soren lifted me up from behind and the midwives pushed my legs up. That's not the position in which we normally have a bowel movement, so that also made it feel weird. Each time I thought that "it" was finally coming out, the midwife told me to stop pushing. About 20 minutes later, when Jacob's head was right in my vaginal opening, they told me to put my hand down and feel it. It was amazing. It was really soft. They said they could see black hair. The midwives whispered something about the baby not having turned its head. This frightened me a bit because I thought there might be something wrong, but all it meant was that the head would be a little harder to give birth to.

By now, I was so tired that I actually fell asleep several times between contractions.

About half an hour after I started pushing, Jacob was born. I don't remember seeing him lifted away from me. Soren said, "It's a boy," and they handed him directly to the pediatrician. I heard him cry, but his cry was brief. Strangely enough, nobody offered to show him to me. Finally, I said, "Can we see him, please?" Apparently most mothers of twins don't want to see baby A until baby B is already born. They let me hold him for a minute. I was completely surprised at the way he looked—not all red and smooshed and wrinkly like everyone said he would, but with a perfectly round head, big blue eyes, and a cleft in his chin just like his father's. He didn't say anything, he just lay perfectly still and rolled his eyes around. (He was probably grateful that I wasn't screaming anymore.)

Then they took him from me and gave him to Soren. The staff was very busy. They broke twin B's water and turned up the oxytocin. The obstetrician said to me, "You let us know when you feel the first contraction." I was rather annoyed at this point, because I felt much too exhausted to go through another half hour of pushing, and well, I was just feeling annoyed at all of them for putting me through this.

What I didn't know until afterward was that baby B arrives like an extra bonus. The birth canal was already opened from giving birth to Jacob's big head. Daniel was slightly smaller, so his head came out on the first push, and with the second push, the rest of him arrived, eight minutes after Jacob. This time I saw them lift him up and hand him over to the pediatrician. Soren exclaimed, "It's another boy!" and that was it.

During my many scans, the doctors had often commented that the babies were lying with their heads right up against each other, and you could see the result of this on Daniel—his head was all dented and his eye was swollen. (Daniel's head straightened out within about three weeks as the doctor had promised it would.) He was also much bloodier than Jacob, but they both had two perfect 10 Apgar scores. Jacob weighed 6 pounds 5 ounces and was 19⅓ inches long. Daniel weighed 6 pounds and was 19 inches long. They were big for twins.

Once the crowd had left the room, we were alone with the midwives again. They reminded Soren to take some pictures, and they asked us the boys' names, promptly learning which one was Jacob and which one was Daniel. I wanted to take a shower and walk around. I had been lying in the bed for as long as I could remember, but I was not allowed to get out of bed except to go to the toilet until we got to the maternity ward.

I had not had an episiotomy, but I had torn a little and they needed to sew me up. The old, tough midwife didn't see any reason to use anesthesia. I just needed a couple of stitches, she said, but I made a big fuss and insisted. After all, hadn't I been through enough already? They had some sort of spray that numbed the area, but I could still feel the needle a few times. I certainly couldn't describe that as painful after experiencing contractions, but I was irritated that I still had to suffer. The midwife trainee was doing it while the older one instructed her. I don't know if that is why it took so long, and I certainly understand that trainees need to get their training somewhere, but I had no more patience and just couldn't wait to get out of that room.

We actually ended up staying there for two more hours because the nurses on the maternity ward were just changing shifts, and they didn't want new patients being brought in until they had gotten organized. They did bring us something to eat and drink and a pay phone so we could call our families.

When they finally came and got us, an orderly wheeled me, on the same bloody bed I had given birth in, to the maternity ward, and Soren walked behind us pushing the boys in their little wheeled bassinet. I sat up in the bed and I remember very clearly two thoughts going through my head: Why in the world does anyone do that more than once? and I'm sure glad I had two. It was much too much work for only one baby!

It was 5:00 p.m. when Soren finally went home, totally exhausted and with a headache. I, on the other hand, had tons of energy and felt just great. I was enormously proud and enormously hungry. And I was treated like a queen on the maternity ward. I was given a single room (all the other mothers had to share), and I had my own changing table (the others used a common room).

That evening, I was really afraid of the boys. I had had practically no experience with children, and I knew nothing about newborns. I was terrified that they might start to cry and I wouldn't know what to do. I didn't dare pick them up. I felt guilty taking one up without the

I KNEW NOTHING ABOUT NEWBORNS. I WAS TERRIFIED THAT THEY MIGHT START TO CRY AND I WOULDN'T KNOW WHAT TO DO. I DIDN'T DARE PICK THEM UP.

other, and besides, they were lying there so nicely, why disturb them? So much for maternal bonding. Daniel, unlike Jacob, had begun making little "eh, eh" sounds as soon as he was born, and he lay there looking at Jacob, making his noises. I caressed his head to comfort him. I kept looking at them. They were beautiful, but I really felt that they were complete strangers. I don't know quite what I had expected, but they had completely surprised me. The whole thing felt very unreal and I wasn't quite convinced they were mine.

In Denmark, you keep your baby with you all the time, but you can ask the nurses to take the baby while you sleep or shower. People who have one baby are allowed to stay in the hospital for up to five days, unless they have had a cesarean, in which case they stay for 10 days. Twins are considered a special situation—you stay until they decide you are ready to go home.

The first evening (and, as it turned out, all the following evenings), the nurses took the boys so I could sleep. They brought them in to me and woke me at night when I had to feed them. They placed a wool-covered tape-recorder that made heartbeat sounds in the bassinet with the babies. In spite of the fact that I had missed an entire night's sleep, I woke up the next morning at 5:30, ravenous, and went to find the boys and the kitchen that always had food available for the new mothers.

The nurse said, "Oh, good, you're awake. They've been wanting to come to you." I remember thinking, Who, me? Why me? I don't know what to do with them. The nurse sensed my feelings. She came back to the room with me and said to the boys, "I think your mother is afraid of you!" and then showed me how to change their diapers. Once we were alone again, I was terrified. I finally got myself to start thinking about the little bit I did know: if they cried, you should check their diaper. If the diaper was dry, they must be either tired or hungry.

I remember the days on the maternity ward as being very long and boring while we waited for Soren to arrive in the evening after work. Luckily the boys didn't do anything to throw me into a panic. I did make one very bad mistake in those first days: I had discovered that my stitches stung when I peed, so I avoided drinking too much liquid, since that just made me have to pee all the time. That was a very bad idea. I was sweating quite a bit, which is normal just after giving birth, and my body needed lots of liquid to replace everything I had lost and was losing (as well as to make milk). As a result of not drinking enough water, I became horribly constipated, and it got worse and worse really quickly because I was so hungry and eating so much all the time. I finally had to get an enema from the nurses. That wasn't fun.

The main concern of the maternity staff was to make sure that my breastfeeding was going well and that the boys did not develop jaundice. As it turned out, the babies did get jaundice, so they had to take blood from their heels for testing twice. It was a heart-wrenching experience for me each time, because the needle obviously hurt them.

On the second day postpartum, I was encouraged to use the breast pump, both to get some of the colostrum out to give to the boys, and to stimulate my milk production. I nursed them during the day, and the nurses used the colostrum in bottles to feed the babies when I was sleeping. Daniel was having trouble getting latched on, and I couldn't figure out how to help him, so the nurses had to help me each time I breast-fed, not just with getting him latched on but with getting the boys in place, and with burping them. It turned out that Jacob was too hungry and needed more than just colostrum, so we finally had to resort to giving him breast milk from another woman (the milk is treated to eliminate contamination with HIV or hepatitis). Finally, on the third day, my milk came in. I was half-sleeping, lying on my stomach, half-sleeping, as I had been instructed to do to help my uterus contract. Suddenly, I became very aware of my breasts. They felt huge and painful. That same day, they informed me, was my "crying" day—the day when I was supposed to go into hormone hell. It actually started the following day, but it lasted for several weeks, not just one day. I've always enjoyed crying—I find it relaxing—so it probably bothered those around me more than it bothered me.

From that point on, I became more and more confident. I actually became so confident that I made the mistake of allowing the babies to breastfeed separately—another recipe for failure for mothers of twins. After one day of that, I realized that it wasn't going to work, and the staff helped me get back on track. It took about an hour to feed them, so if I didn't feed them at the same time, I could wind up feeding them all day long. I used a big half-doughnut-shaped cushion propped up with pillows, and the boys lay on their sides with their legs under my arms and heads to my breasts. They switched breasts at each feeding. Whenever one was hungry, we'd wake the other one and force him to eat, too. We came home a week after the day they were born, once their jaundice was under control and they had begun to gain weight.

During that week on the maternity ward, incredible maternal feelings of overwhelming love and the desire to protect the babies arose in me. By the end of the week, I knew why people "do that" again and again, and I also knew that I, too, wanted to experience it again—not anytime soon, but definitely again in my lifetime. Giving birth was absolutely the most difficult physical thing I've ever accomplished, but I was incredibly proud of myself for doing it. Now I know how strong I am. It was without a doubt the most amazing day in my life.

Fifty Minutes in a Birthing Center

*Mary and her husband, Thomas, are both computer
systems administrators who live in Queens, New York.
Their baby was born in a Manhattan birthing center that is
affiliated with a hospital. They were both 29 years
old at the time of Nicholas's birth.*

I was very active before getting pregnant and continued to exercise
until it became uncomfortable to do so. I swam throughout my
pregnancy, worked out with prenatal exercise videos, and lifted
weights until I was eight months along. During the last two months, all
I could do aerobically was swim, because I had begun to experience pain
in the ligaments supporting the uterus.

On Wednesday, February 22, 1995, I spent the day setting up some
new computer equipment in our home office so I could work from home
after the baby was born. In the evening, my husband, Thomas, and I
went to the gym, and I went swimming. It was four days before my due
date, and I was having more contractions than usual. Usually, I'd have

four or five Braxton Hicks contractions per day, always at different times, but this day I had many more.

Most days I swam between 30 and 50 laps. That evening, I had painless contractions throughout my swim and felt uncomfortable, but I pressed on and finished 40 laps. The swim helped ease a slight backache, but the contractions kept coming, one after the other, and they started coming more frequently, about every seven minutes. After our swim, we went home and had salmon and vegetables for dinner.

That night, I was not able to sleep as well as usual. The contractions continued throughout the night, a little more intense, but still at the same rate and not yet painful. I got up several times to go to the bathroom, which provided no relief since I kept feeling pressure on my bladder. But so far, there was no pain at all, just discomfort in my entire abdominal area and in a small section of my lower back.

The next morning, I kept having the same contractions but I told Thomas to go ahead and go to work. I figured if it was a false alarm, there was no sense in getting him all worried about it. I told him I'd call him when I needed him. After he left, I worked some more on setting up the new computer equipment and made some phone calls. All the while I was aware of the incessant contractions, but they still didn't hurt.

At about 10:00 a.m., I went to the bathroom and saw some faint traces of blood on the tissue, watery and pink. I figured this must be the "bloody show." Could this be it? I called a friend who was supposed to stop by that day, to tell her not to come over; I had a feeling I'd be busy. I also called Connie, my best friend, who lives in Cleveland and is a doula, to tell her what was happening. She thought it sounded like the beginning of labor. So I called the maternity center and described what had been happening; Marcy, the midwife on duty, told me to continue my day as usual, to relax, eat, and drink well. I remembered that we had made plans for that evening with friends, so I canceled them. Then I called Thomas and told him he should come home.

By 11:00 a.m., the contractions had started to feel like menstrual cramps on either side of my uterus, where I imagine the fallopian tubes to be. So far, everything I was feeling was in the front part of my abdomen. I poured myself a glass of red wine, as my midwife had suggested, and began timing the contractions. I called my two sisters, my parents, and a couple of friends to let them know what was happening. The contractions were coming about every eight minutes, and lasting 30 seconds. They continued like that for a couple of hours. The wine helped me relax.

At 1:00 p.m., it began to hurt a little. The crampy feeling was getting strong, even painful, exactly like strong menstrual cramps on both sides, in the lower abdomen. I tried my breathing exercises, and they helped. I inhaled slowly through my nose and exhaled very slowly through my mouth. Around this time, Thomas got home. Since I was managing fine, he decided to clean the kitchen floor while I halfheartedly watched television and did my breathing exercises.

My brother lives about five minutes from the maternity center in Manhattan, so we had planned to spend some of my labor time at his apartment. From where we live in Queens, it can take anywhere from 20 to 45 minutes to get to the birthing center, or even longer if traffic is really bad. It was the middle of February, so I was also worried about the possibility of snow. But I thought we could wait a while and leave when the program I was watching was over.

By the middle of the program, however, the contractions had become so strong that my breathing exercises were no longer very effective. Now the only positions that were comfortable for me were standing up or sitting down and leaning back against a pillow. Anything else made the pain worse. I was pretty quiet, unless the contraction was a really painful one. Then I groaned.

At about 3:30 p.m., we decided to go into the city. I put on my coat and sneakers, and we headed out with our overnight bag and the baby's car seat. I walked ever so slowly down one flight of stairs and out through our lobby. It was drizzling but not too cold. Maybe snow would not be a problem after all.

I felt better sitting in the car. Some of the contractions were very strong and painful, but they still lasted only about 40 to 45 seconds, with about a four-minute break in between. I did some breathing exercises, but they weren't helping much.

We reached my brother's apartment sometime around 4:30. I hardly remember the ride at all, but I know that we took the Triborough Bridge and that traffic was mercifully light. Thomas dropped me off in front of Bill's building and went to find a parking space. I breathed through a couple more contractions while standing outside Bill's door, fumbling with the key.

It was a relief to be in his quiet apartment. I settled down on the bed and leaned against a giant stuffed bear, which surprisingly was very comfortable. I started watching television again, but I couldn't figure

out how to change the channel, so I wound up with an afternoon talk
show about men who think they're God's gift to women! This was not
what I expected exactly during labor, but the contractions were already
so intense that I really didn't care. In the meantime, Thomas came in
with some Chinese food; he was starving. I ate a little cereal and drank
some apple juice, but it was hard to eat; I was slightly nauseated and the
apple juice made the nausea worse. I had eaten very little all day; probably just a banana and some bread, plus the red wine.

Over the next two hours, I tried to get comfortable. Standing up to
relieve the pain didn't work. I found that the best positions for me were
leaning back against the bear or sitting on the toilet. I drew a warm bath
but never got in the tub because I didn't have the energy to take my
clothes off. Thomas did his best to help me continue the breathing exercises. Between contractions, I fell into a trancelike sleep, which
helped me conserve energy. The phone rang a lot but we let the answering machine get the calls, except once, when we could hear it was
Bill. He wanted to talk to me but I couldn't talk. Then it occurred to
me that if I was unable to talk during a contraction, perhaps it was time
to go to the maternity center. We called there at 7:00 p.m. and my midwife, Marcy, could tell from my voice that it was indeed time, so we
headed over.

I thought I could walk to the car, a couple of blocks away. I had two
contractions in the elevator of Bill's building, then another once we
were out on the street. We walked very slowly toward the car. We had
to stop several times by a tree or a parking meter so I could lean against
and breathe through a contraction. It was quite a long two blocks, but

we made it to the car. Again, I found that sitting down offered relief.

We arrived at the maternity center at about 7:30. I had to stop on the steps going up to the side entrance, for another contraction. Thomas wanted me to get onto level ground, but I just stood there on a step. A woman named Ernie opened the door and let me in while Thomas went to park the car. Ernie seemed very strong and not at all surprised by my appearance. Somehow, her strength transferred to me and made me feel a little better. I took off my coat and Marcy told me to give her a urine sample, which I did. The urine test indicated that I was dehydrated, so Marcy ordered me to drink the bottle of Gatorade that Thomas had brought with him. Next, Marcy did a quick exam. She said, "This is great, Mary, you're 10 centimeters dilated!" I was ready to go into the birthing room and have the baby! We couldn't believe it.

The birthing room was cozy, decorated in pale greens and soft whites, with floral curtains. I remember the bed had a light green sheet on it. There were lamps and medical supplies, but the dominating feature was the big tub in the middle of the room, like a Jacuzzi. Once inside the room, I took off all my clothing and jewelry and immediately got into a squatting position next to the bathtub. The feel of the cool tile was soothing. As soon as I got into this position, my water broke. It really felt like something popping. Someone asked if I wanted to draw a bath and I said yes. As the water was running, I moved a few feet away to lean against a birthing stool, which allowed me to remain in a squatting position without becoming too tired. Thomas pulled up a chair behind me and held me under my arms. He also played some music we had brought with us.

I think I began pushing as soon as my water broke, about 7:45. Marcy told me to just go with the pushing, to push the baby out. Until now, I'd been pretty quiet, but each time I pushed, I could not help but scream as loud as I've ever screamed in my life. In fact, it was as if the sound was not coming from my voice, but from the depths of somewhere else, almost an "out of body" experience. The pushing was an incredible force against my whole body. About half an hour later, with me still in the same squatting position, leaning against the stool and Thomas, I heard Marcy say, "This baby has a lot of hair!" She had me feel the baby's head as he came out. All the while, Marcy had been applying warm compresses and oil to my perineum so that he eased out gently.

> EACH TIME I PUSHED, I COULD NOT HELP BUT SCREAM AS LOUD AS I'VE EVER SCREAMED IN MY LIFE. THE SOUND CAME FROM THE DEPTHS OF SOMEWHERE ELSE, ALMOST AN "OUT OF BODY" EXPERIENCE.

On February 23, 1995, at 8:20 p.m., only 50 minutes after we'd arrived, Nicholas was born. I reached down and lifted him up just as he entered the world. He felt very warm and slippery, and I looked at him and saw his beautiful face. I suspected he was a boy, and when I looked at him, I saw that indeed he was. I held him close to my heart as Thomas hugged both of us.

Marcy swabbed him down a little, then cut the umbilical cord. The cord, his source of life for so long, was very thick and twisted. One more push and the afterbirth was expelled. Ordinarily I would have thought it was very strange looking, but in this context it was interesting. Then Marcy quickly diapered Nicholas and I stood up. I looked down and my stomach was almost flat. I felt an odd, unaccustomed emptiness as I realized my stomach and lungs suddenly had some space again; I could immediately breathe more easily, but I also felt light-headed and my heart was beating very fast.

I lay down on the bed with Thomas and Nicholas. I had torn just a little, and Marcy repaired me with a couple of stitches. She injected me with a local anesthetic, so the stitching didn't hurt at all.

I could not take my eyes off the baby. I put him to my breast, and he suckled immediately, making Thomas and me realize we were also really hungry. About an hour later, Thomas went out and got us some food. When he came back, the three of us were left alone in the cozy, softly lit room. I was able to take a shower and freshen up. I felt a little shaky, especially my legs, and the newly empty feeling in my upper abdomen was uncomfortable. My heart rate was still elevated.

As we all were getting used to each other, we listened to music and rested. It was raining outside. Listening to the rain against the windowpanes soothed me. Soon Thomas and Nicholas fell asleep. While I watched the two of them, I saw clearly how much they looked alike.

I could hear the woman in the next birthing room going through all that I had just gone through. I tried to encourage her with my thoughts. (Her baby was finally born early the next morning, just before we left.)

During the course of the night, he was weighed and measured, and his footprints were recorded. I was surprised at how big he was: 8 pounds, 9 ounces, and 21 inches long. Before we left, the midwife swabbed him off (not really a bath), and gave him Vitamin K and eye ointment. We filled out all of Nicholas's papers. Before we left we also scheduled an appointment with a nurse who would come to our home the next day to give us a 24-hour checkup, and one with our pediatrician for Nicholas's first examination.

The next morning, at 7:00 a.m., we swaddled the baby, put him in his car seat, and left the city with Nicholas. I sat in the back seat of the car, marveling at his tiny face. He was content as we crossed the bridge that rainy February day and headed home to begin our new life as a family.

The Case of the Unopened Suitcase

Jennifer, 27, was a tutor and substitute elementary school teacher when her first child was born in a hospital in Durham, North Carolina. Her husband, John, a graduate student and social science researcher at a local university, was also 27 years old.

I was a day overdue at my last doctor's appointment. The doctor said that after a week or so, an induction would be considered and she would want to schedule a non-stress test at that time, but meanwhile, we would just "wait and see." She also told me that if I had any signs of labor, I should phone the hospital immediately for advice.

Four days later, on February 29, at around noon, I went into labor on my own. My contractions began 11 minutes apart and were so strong I had to lie down. Unlike the tightening of the Braxton Hicks contractions I'd had for the last month, which were not painful or even uncomfortable, these contractions felt like *very* bad cramps. They were painful and uncomfortable from the very beginning, and were centered

153

around the area of my belly button. The Braxton Hicks contractions had involved a painless tightening of my entire stomach.

At first I thought something might be wrong, since the cramping was so intense and painful. Clearly different from the Braxton Hicks. So I called the hospital and spoke to a resident, who advised that I stay home. It was about 1:00 p.m. She said since it was my first birth, I probably had hours to go. But by the end of our phone conversation, the contractions were five minutes apart.

My mother had had short labors. She had about six hours of labor with me. At the time, she was one of the first women in this country to have an epidural. They had given it to her immediately upon her arrival at the hospital. Since she was dilated only 2 centimeters, the epidural probably slowed her down. She said she read magazines for five hours, and then the nurses came in and told her it was time to push. My brother was born after less than two hours of labor, and my dad, a doctor, couldn't be reached in time to drive my mom to the hospital. Luckily, they lived only two blocks away, so she walked over, carrying her suitcase. Dad arrived in time to grab a wheelchair and meet her at the sidewalk and wheel her in. She was taken straight to the delivery room, given a spinal block, and an hour later, she had my brother.

My mom's and my pregnancies had been similar, so I had assumed we might also have similar labors. Since my contractions were already five minutes apart after only an hour, and they were so intense I was doubling over, I told my husband, John, "You've got to get me to the hospital before I can't walk." Luckily he was working at home that day and we were able to leave for the hospital right away.

When we arrived, at approximately 1:45 p.m., I told John, "I know I'll need your help getting in." I was still doubling over with each contraction and I didn't want to wait for a wheelchair. The hospital, which is a teaching hospital, is so large and the building so complicated, I thought it would be faster if we just walked in. I was convinced it would take twice as long to wait for someone to bring out a wheelchair. So he had to hold onto me and help me up the stairs. He left our car with my suitcase in it in the hospital driveway drop-off zone, thinking he would go back to get the suitcase and move the car while I was checking in and getting settled into the room.

But it turned out things were progressing so quickly that the nurses wouldn't let him leave. They wanted him to stay and help me get to my room and change into my gown. My first internal exam showed that I had already dilated 4 centimeters. The intern said she would go get my doctor, and a nurse placed an external monitor on me.

I had considered an epidural ahead of time and had listened carefully during the childbirth classes to the explanation of the procedure, though I thought I would wait and see if I needed it. After I arrived, I knew I wouldn't be walking around or taking a shower for relief. The nurses were trying to get me to do the breathing exercises, but I couldn't do them. My contractions were so intense, I couldn't concentrate on anything. I realized I couldn't be helpful in any way, and I was worried that at this rate, I wouldn't be able to be helpful at the delivery stage either, so I immediately asked for the epidural. This hospital has a dedicated ob-gyn anesthesiologist, so you are not sharing the anesthesiologist with the surgery department, and he was able to come immediately.

The nurses began to prepare me the minute I asked for the epidural. My husband signed the permission letters, and the nurses got an IV started on me. By this time, both the anesthesiologist and my own doctor had arrived. The anesthesiologist turned out to be the same one who had led our prenatal class's epidural presentation. Forty-five minutes later, when I was already 7 centimeters dilated, the epidural was started and immediately I relaxed. Although I still felt the pressure of the contractions, now I could enjoy and participate in the experience. I became much more friendly.

WAITING FOR THE EPIDURAL, I WOULDN'T HAVE CARED IF I WAS IN YANKEE STADUIM, AS LONG AS SOMEONE WAS PREPARING MY PAIN RELIEF.

My dilation was so rapid, students had been coming to observe me. At one point, there were about a dozen people in the room. This didn't bother me: I was pretty used to being observed. As a college student, I was always asked in the on-campus clinic if someone could observe my routine checkups. Plus, since my dad is a doctor, the idea was not foreign to me. The students were all quite unobtrusive. Besides, while waiting for the epidural, I wouldn't have cared if I was in Yankee Stadium, as long as someone was preparing my pain relief. During the insertion of the epidural the doctor was making wordy explanations to the students, while I was thinking to myself, "Quick, stick that needle in!"

Meanwhile, my mother had driven in from two hours away, and stuck her head in the door and said, "I'm here, is there anything I can do?" John and I said, in unison, "Please move our car!" When she got to the driveway, a ticket was on the windshield, and the tow truck was backing up. Fortunately, when the tow truck driver heard my mother's story, he removed the equipment. My mom moved the car to the parking lot and finally brought in my suitcase. But she forgot it in the waiting room because by the time she had returned with it, it was time for me to push and she had to rush upstairs to be with us.

This was at about 4:00 p.m. The nurse who had been watching the monitor told me it was time to push. She was a wonderful nurse and helped me immensely. She asked if I could feel my contractions. I could, but only as a kind of pressure. So she quizzed me. She said, "Tell me when the next one starts and when it stops." I did so. She said, "Okay, you are agreeing with the monitor. So go ahead and push with the next one and I'll tell you when to stop." I pushed for 20 minutes, with my terrific nurse saying encouraging things the whole time. I could feel the pressure of my daughter's head when she crowned, but absolutely no pain. Grace Carol was born after four and a half hours of labor, at 4:19 p.m. She was 7 pounds, 3 ounces, and 19 inches long. She was placed at my breast before the cord was even cut.

Later, when my husband finally went back downstairs, he found my suitcase still sitting in the waiting room. Ironically, even though I had packed that suitcase when I was seven months pregnant and had filled it with every labor aid I'd ever read about or could think of, in the end, it was never even opened!

I had always thought the quick check-out times for new mothers were criminal, but I found that after 24 hours, I was more than ready to go home, eat some good food, and let my mom take care of me.

I'd tell other mothers in labor for the first time to trust their instincts and be flexible. I had had all sorts of daydreams about what my labor would be like: I would phone my husband to tell him it had started, then I'd walk the dog. I'd have plenty of time, since I had already packed my suitcase . . .

Also, women should make sure their husbands take great mental notes on everything that happens. I grilled mine later on the details that were a blur to me. Thank goodness he remembered.

Long Labor, Quick Delivery

David was born with the assistance of his father and a midwife
in his parents' home, a modern house clinging to a rocky hillside
in a subdivision outside Victoria, British Columbia. Kate was
29 years old, and Graeme was 40 at the time of their son's birth.
They are both computer systems professionals, so naturally,
they posted the story of David's birth on their Web site.

GRAEME: David William was born Friday, September 15, at 5:30 a.m. He weighed 8.5 pounds and was 22 inches long. His eyes are dark blue and he has fairish hair; no saying how he will end up yet.

The total labor time was about 30 hours, although everything seemed to happen in the last three hours. Kate started early labor at 11:00 p.m. on Wednesday and had contractions as close as seven minutes for a few hours during the night. The contractions eased off during the day on Thursday and then started to pick up again in the evening. Up to this point, the contractions had been of varying degrees, some much more intense than others. It was difficult for me at times. Kate would ask me to press on her lower back to help relieve the pain and I would think, Okay, now I know what I have to do to help. But as the next contraction started, I would put my hand on her lower back, only to have her push my hand away saying, "No, don't do that."

KATE: It was really unpredictable, and a small, sane corner in my brain knew that I wasn't making things easy for Graeme, but the truth is there was no single thing he could reliably do from contraction to contraction to help me. We had to make it up as we went along.

That first night, the contractions were regular, seven to eight minutes apart, but otherwise unimpressive. During the next day, they remained at the same rate, but became increasingly uncomfortable.

GRAEME: We worked with a team of midwives, Kim and Luba. Kim visited in the afternoon and again in the evening, but was of the opinion that the birth was quite a ways off, perhaps not even until Saturday. The cervix was still well back and had not dilated. We didn't tell Kate, as she was getting a bit fatigued by this point and the thought of another two days of labor would have been rather disheartening for her to say the least.

KATE: Oh, yes . . .

GRAEME: Kim also thought that the baby had gone posterior (his back to Kate's back) despite having been in a nice anterior position for the last couple of months. She gave Kate a sedative to help her sleep and then left at about 9:00 Thursday evening. Much of the pain Kate was having was due to her back labor.

KATE: This part was pretty rough. I knew about the baby being posterior and was digging in for the long run, but each contraction was hurting, and we'd already been at this for 24 hours. As I drifted in and out of sleep that night, the contractions slowly accelerated to a frequency of four to five minutes. Not having dilated at all in 24 hours, what happened next was so sudden that we weren't mentally prepared. We believed we were still in prodromal labor right up until it became amply clear that David was just about to be born. Meanwhile, I was still dreading another day or two like this . . .

GRAEME: The sedative did not work and at 2:30 a.m. I called Kim to tell her. At this time, the contractions were still about the same as they had been when Kim left that evening, so we felt there had probably been little progress and I agreed to call her again in two hours with an update.

A half hour later, Kate became aware that something had changed. After the birth, Kim surmised that this was when the baby had turned to an anterior position.

KATE: All this is with 20/20 hindsight, of course. But yes, at 3:00 a.m., I felt the baby flip around. I had a very odd feeling, like a "blooop," and then the contractions *really* hit. They became double-peaked with hardly a break between them. I got up on my hands and knees in bed. During a contraction, I rocked back and forth, and yelled. (I was quite hoarse the next day.) In between them, I moaned. I would just finish with one con-traction, when *bam*, along would come the next. I felt helpless. Each time I would think, I can't do this, and then, each time, I did it.

Eventually, I needed to go to the bathroom. Sitting on the toilet felt so good, I began to alternate between rocking on the bed, and sit-ting on the toilet.

> **YOU JUST DON'T MESS AROUND WITH THE URGE TO PUSH. IT'S ALMOST IRRESISTIBLE, DEEPLY ANIMAL, AND WILD.**

I was, at this point, in very late first stage labor (fully dilated), probably in transition, but I couldn't bring myself to believe it, since we had made so little progress over the last day. I was hurting a lot. When my mom phoned to check in at about 4:30 a.m., I wondered if the neigh-bors had called the cops on us. I was howl-ing with the pain.

GRAEME: At 4:00 a.m., the contractions started getting closer and a lot more in-tense, and during one of her toilet sits, Kate was having very strong urges to push the baby out. We both thought that this was far too early to be pushing so we tried to control her breathing to counteract the urge.

KATE: Despair was setting in on my part. My mental state said, "Sorry, girl, but this is probably much too early, and you're just going to have to pant through these for another day or two . . . " But I'm here to tell you that you just don't mess around with the urge to push. It's almost irresistible, deeply animal, and wild. It takes a stronger head than I have to be able to override the animal brain at this point of labor.

GRAEME: At 4:30, I called Kim, and when she heard what was happening she decided to come 'round immediately. Five minutes later, just after she climbed back into bed, Kate's water broke. For the first time, we knew things were far more advanced than we thought.

The first midwife arrived at 4:55 a.m. and after a quick examination, she discovered that the baby was already crowning . . .

KATE: I couldn't believe it!

GRAEME: . . . So she immediately phoned her partner to come over, and then started getting all her equipment set up for the birth. At about 5:20 a.m. the head was fully out and Kim tried to get Kate to slow down, as she felt the baby was coming a little too quickly. Kim wanted the muscles to stretch a bit more to prevent any tearing.

KATE: It took Kim in my face to get me to hold off. I'm amazed at how "far away" I was while in late labor. There's clearly an art to communicating with a laboring woman, and I'm really impressed at how Kim managed to get me back under control. The poor woman was trying to deal with a baby that was about to pop out of one end of me, and me, mentally somewhere else, trying my best to push the baby out as quickly as possible. She simultaneously put one hand on the baby's head, to keep track of its progress, and put her nose inches from mine. She made eye contact and said very, very clearly, distinctly, and coolly, "Kate, you have to stop *now*." I panted in reply. So she said, "Kate, slow down *now*." The combination of having her face so close to mine and her repeated use of my name finally got through to me and enabled me to focus and to slow down. With Kim's assistance, I was able to ease the baby out.

GRAEME: It really was amazing to see that little head sticking out from between Kate's legs. By getting Kate to hold back as best she could, Kim gave the perineum time to stretch a bit more, thus reducing Kate's tear. After six or seven minutes she asked Kate to start pushing again, and two minutes later, there was David William. I was impressed by how small he was and by his cone-shaped head. Even though he was now right there in front of me, it was still hard to grasp that this *person* had been growing and developing inside Kate for the last nine months. But here he was. We now had a baby.

KATE: For me, it was bliss. As soon as the head was out, the driving need to push, and the pain, faded very fast. I went from fighting Kim when she wanted me to *not* push, to having trouble gathering enough of myself to push the shoulders out. I have tremendous respect for women who birth with anesthesia in place, which blocks the involuntary pushing feeling. I think it would have taken twice as long for him to have been born if I'd had to push only when I was told to.

GRAEME: Luba, Kim's partner, joined us just seconds after the birth, having run every red light between her house and ours. Kim immediately placed the baby on Kate's stomach. One of my most vivid impressions is from this moment. At the first sight of her son, Kate broke into a great big smile. It still amazes me that within seconds of giving birth, a mother forgets about the pain.

David gave a couple of short splutters, and then he was off and running. He did not require any stimulation. As soon as David started breathing, the cord stopped pulsating and the midwives clamped, and then cut the cord. Within another five minutes, Kate had delivered the placenta intact. Then it was a case of cleaning David,

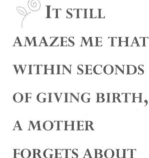 **IT STILL AMAZES ME THAT WITHIN SECONDS OF GIVING BIRTH, A MOTHER FORGETS ABOUT THE PAIN.**

although he was actually very clean, a lot less messy than I had expected. One of my biggest fears had been about the blood. I do not respond well to the sight of it. But David emerged so clean and Kate bled so little that I was fine. I had survived the birth without keeling over.

KATE: After I had delivered the placenta, Kim saw that the rapidity of the birth had indeed caused a slight tear in my perineum, so she and Luba put in a couple of stitches. By the third day after the birth, I was already over the hump with the sore bottom thing . . . a ginger and comfrey root decoction applied as a compress was wonderful.

GRAEME: Once things had calmed down and we had time to reflect, the midwives believed that Kate probably went from zero dilation to full dilation in less than two hours.

KATE: Yes, zero to zero dilation in 28 hours, zero to 10 in two. Kim has warned me that if I do this again, my midwife and I should be ready for a fast labor, as long as the kid's pointing in the right direction . . .

GRAEME: The movement Kate had felt at 3:00 a.m. was the baby turning, and this had allowed the cervix to finally come forward and dilate. The rest is history.

This experience had taught me several things. The first is that no matter how well you know your partner, be prepared for that knowledge to go right out the window during labor. Things can change from minute to minute. During one contraction, she will ask you to do something, so you think, "Aha! This is what she wants." With the next contraction you repeat your action only to have it met by a mouthful of abuse, and you realize that is no longer what she needs. Be prepared to go with the flow.

Second, for those like me who worry about fainting during the birth, the process is not as bloody as you might expect. Even if it is, you are so preoccupied with caring for your mate, you have no time to think about such things.

Third, prepare yourself for the sight of your mate in pain, and at times, considerable pain. Remember that the pain does pass, and that it's part and parcel of birth. Finally, your mate may have little recollection of her experience. She may ask you to relate what happened at the various stages. It can turn out that you have worse memories than she does!

KATE: In the end, a Yuppie, type-A personality control freak like me learned to let go and to let it happen. We did a lot better when we stopped timing and carefully comparing contractions to the What-Happens-in-Labor charts, and just got on with having the baby.

The late first stage was liberating for me. I just did what my body commanded. Rock? Okay. Toilet? Okay. Yell? Okay. Without my consciously doing so, I did what I had to do to get the baby born.

I think laboring woman's greatest privilege is to be arbitrary and capricious, to let go of being "a good girl." For me, a skillful, sensitive midwife stands back unless intervention is clearly indicated, as it was when my baby came bombing out.

I'm a big fan of home births now. If we'd been planning on a hospital birth, I certainly would have been sent home if we'd gone to the hospital any time in those first 28 hours, and we just might not have gotten back in time during those last two. Graeme and David and I have been able to nest together and get to know each other in the peace and quiet of our own house and our own bed. Luba comes by daily to check on us. I wish we had a health care system that could guarantee *all* moms the postpartum home support we're getting, whether they give birth at home or in a hospital.

GRAEME: As the proud father, I just have to add that I think David is the cutest baby I have ever seen!

Don't Be a Martyr

*Caron is a film executive and writer who lives in
New York City with her two children. She had her first child
in a hospital when she was 24 years old. Her then-husband,
Eddie, was 26 years old and a baker.*

He's big now—6 feet, 2 inches at 15 years old—and he was big then. On a tranquil Palm Sunday, April 8, 1979, at 7:10 in the morning, my first child was born. Lonn weighed in at 9 pounds, 4½ ounces, and he was 21 inches long. He was beautiful, and his hair was perfectly styled. Mine was a mess.

My pregnancy was uneventful, except for the amount of weight I gained: 45 pounds! I tipped the scales at 180 the day of delivery. For me, the most memorable and sobering revelation of Lamaze class was when the teacher told us, "Don't expect to wear your regular jeans home from the hospital." I couldn't wear my regular jeans until my son was seven months old. And a week after I finally managed to zip them up while lying on the bed, I found out I was pregnant with my daughter!

I went into labor on my due date, April 7. At about 10:00 that morning, I felt my first contraction. It felt like a menstrual cramp, or like the belt on a stationary bicycle being tightened around the wheel as the tension increases (the wheel being my mammoth stomach). The first one lasted only a few seconds. It was actually what I thought it would feel like: a wave of seismic activity taking place inside me. It wasn't terribly painful at first, but it was intense.

I called the doctor and he said we should come right over. My then-husband, Eddie, wanted to be very involved in the birth experience and had taken Lamaze classes with me. On the way to the doctor's office, about 20 minutes after the first contraction, I felt another one. This one had more edge than the first. Eddie reminded me to breathe, like I had learned in the Lamaze class, and I did. The breathing doesn't take the pain away, but the counting and the holding and the pushing out the stress does distract you from feeling the pain.

The doctor examined me and told us I was partially dilated, that we should go home and rest and that I should not eat any solid foods. He said we should call him when the contractions were five minutes apart or if my water broke. (It never did break by itself. The doctor broke it later in the hospital.) He also warned me that as the contractions came closer together, they would become more fierce.

As usual, I was starving, so, disregarding the doctor's orders, I insisted that Eddie take me for Chinese food, and he indulged me. By now, the contractions were coming every 15 minutes or so but because they didn't last very long, maybe only 15 to 30 seconds, I was still able to enjoy my meal.

At about 10:30 that evening, my contractions began coming every five minutes. We called the doctor and told him we were on our way to the hospital. I was feeling a little tired but was holding up very well. I am a sturdy, solidly built woman, and I'm not a big kvetcher. I also had youth on my side. I was a month shy of 25 years old, a mere child myself.

On the way to Jamaica Hospital in Queens, I was flush with exhilaration and anxiety. My train of thought went something like this: was the pain going to be more than I could bear? Would my baby be perfect? If something were physically wrong with my child, of course I would still love the baby, but how would I deal with it? If it was a boy, would we name him Lonn or Luke? A girl we thought would be Lara. We needed a name that began with "L." In the Jewish tradition, we were naming our child after Eddie's grandmother, Lena, who had passed away five years before.

We checked in to the hospital and I was wheeled into the delivery room. The doctor on duty came in and told me that my obstetrician would be there soon. I was now 7 centimeters dilated and the contractions were getting rough. I was breathing, and Eddie was holding my hand and being very loving, supportive, and just so "there." I suddenly felt the urge to move my bowels and asked the doctor if I could get up. He said this was not a good idea, that he would bring me a bedpan. And then I had to have a bowel movement in front of Eddie, the doctor, and the nurses. It was profoundly embarrassing. However, considering the various and sundry smells and fluids oozing and dripping out of me—the blood, sweat, and tears (of happiness)—and my wide-open legs, the bedpan merely set the stage for an early morning of no shame.

My doctor arrived about 4:00 a.m. and I was so happy to see him. I had thought he would have come right after I was admitted. The hospital's doctors, of course, are well-trained and competent, but I felt more comfortable with my own. He felt around inside me and said things were looking fine. I was doing pretty well at this point. The pain of the contractions was vivid but not excruciating. I heard a woman in the next room screaming and thought maybe I was being spared.

However, an hour later I knew I was not. By 5:00 a.m., the inside of my body felt like a war zone. Now the contractions were about two minutes apart and were lasting longer, almost a minute, and each one felt like an 18-wheel truck was rolling over me, through me, and under me.

The other pearl of wisdom our Lamaze instructor had given us was, "If you need some painkillers to take the edge off the pain, take them. It's still considered natural childbirth. Don't be a martyr." Well, I couldn't handle the pain and asked the good doctor for some drugs. He ordered something to be given intra-

OUR LAMAZE INSTRUCTOR HAD TOLD US, "IF YOU NEED PAINKILLERS TO TAKE THE EDGE OFF THE PAIN, TAKE THEM. DON'T BE A MARTYR."

venously. It seemed to have an immediate effect and, as promised, it took the edge off my pain. I felt a little high.

Sometime after 6:00 a.m. it was time to push. This was the hardest part. I didn't know the baby was so big. I only knew that pushing was painful. However, the pain was mitigated both by the drug and by the knowledge that finally, after nine months of pregnancy and all this pain and breathing and pushing, we would see the results of my labor, our work of art. So I kept pushing, and the doctor kept saying, "You're doing great, you're doing great, I see the head! It's crowning!" I thought just then that I would faint from joy. And the good doctor said, "Come on Caron, one more big push!" I inhaled and exhaled and ordered my muscles with every ounce of strength I could muster up to push out. I felt my baby's head coming through my vagina and then just whooshing out of me. They all said, "It's a boy." He looked pretty perfect to me and I started crying and hugging my doctor and my husband.

With a Little Help from My Friends

Krystie was 26 and single, working as a data entry clerk,
when she had her son at home in Manhattan
with the assistance of a midwife
and six of her friends.

I had decided to have my baby at home and had found a wonderful, very down-to-earth certified nurse-midwife to attend the birth. She screened me for all the likely risks. When she measured my pelvis, she told me that if the baby went over 10 pounds before birth, I'd have to deliver by cesarean. But that was a remote possibility. The scariest thing that happened was that one day during my eighth month, I began bleeding at work. At the hospital, they said my placenta had torn slightly, but the baby was fine. I had to spend the next few weeks in bed.

My due date came and went. Ten days later, I went into labor at about 4:00 a.m. I was awakened by the contractions, and I knew it was labor because my mother had told me that labor pains felt like strong menstrual cramps at first. The contractions started at five-minute intervals and they never slowed down or stopped. I tried to sleep, but it was difficult. At around 8:00 a.m., I called the friends who planned to be with me for the birth, and they started coming over.

My midwife had warned me that it would be a long, painful labor because the baby's head was engaged in a posterior position, facing front (most babies face back). She said that instead of the baby's forehead inserting itself slowly into the cervix like a wedge, the back of the baby's head would hit the cervix bluntly, like a battering ram, with each contraction. She was right. It hurt intensely with each contraction, to the point where normally I would have begged for it to stop; but I hadn't realized how tough I was or how much I could handle. I had to keep focused on the fact that my body was not being damaged, and remind myself that this was a natural process that would lead to my baby coming out. I made myself accept the pain as necessary.

I HADN'T REALIZED HOW TOUGH I WAS OR HOW MUCH I COULD HANDLE.

After 16 hours, thinking I'd had painful, productive labor, I called my midwife saying I was sure that things had progressed pretty far. My mother, who'd been in labor for 36 hours when she had me, had often told me that her labor pains weren't much worse than heavy menstrual cramps. (My dad confirmed that Mom never even raised her voice during the worst of the pain.) The pain I had already experienced seemed worse than that. But I was still joking with my friends about how glad I was not to have to pack a bag or to get dressed and go to the hospital in the middle of the night.

My midwife arrived with her big bag of equipment, put on her rubber gloves, and measured my cervix. It had dilated only 3 centimeters. She had me take a warm bath, and within a couple of hours, I had dilated to 6 centimeters. The pain became incredible, but I was determined to stick with it. The contractions felt like I was being hit in the stomach with a baseball bat. But I was certain that any painkillers I took would reduce the strength of the contractions, prolong the labor, and possibly enter the baby's bloodstream, so I declined them. I didn't want to give up and go to a hospital unless my midwife felt it was medically necessary. However, I did give up our family stoicism at that point and yelled whenever I felt like it. That felt much better.

I had six friends with me, and I needed them all. My midwife wanted me to drink and eat at least once an hour, so someone had to keep a chart of that. Someone else had to keep a chart of my contractions. Someone else had to hold me upright or help me use the toilet, or entertain or commiserate with me. Whenever one of them left to attend to her own family, she was sorely missed.

Meanwhile, I was used to being a considerate hostess, and in between contractions, I kept trying to fix people food and offer them drinks. I even apologized for the mess the apartment was in. Finally, one friend, a lay midwife from Italy, told me I had to stop thinking of everyone as my guest and remember that they were there to wait on me. To make things easier for me, she went through the apartment and put a layer of plastic and absorbent pads over every flat surface. She also put layers of waterproof pads and sheet sets on the bed, so that we could just pull off a soiled layer and not have to change the bed. I felt well taken care of, but guilty watching her work.

Pain is very transforming. After 24 hours had passed, I became first petulant, then downright mean. And yet all my friends indulged me. It was great. At one point during a really heavy contraction, someone started making droning noises, as if she expected me to "sound" with her. I told her to shut up. Normally, I would never have been so rude, but I figured I could apologize later.

One of the most effective ways I found for managing the pain was to visualize it as an ocean wave that crested in the middle of a contraction and then fell. I imagined myself as a swimmer in stormy breakers. I kept telling myself that as soon as the pain felt its worst, it meant the worst was already over. Then whoever was coaching me at that moment would remind me to focus on the upcoming pain-free minutes and would check the clock to tell me how much time I had left in the contraction.

I IMAGINED MYSELF AS A SWIMMER IN STORMY BREAKERS. I KEPT TELLING MYSELF THAT AS SOON AS THE PAIN FELT ITS WORST, IT MEANT THE WORST WAS ALREADY OVER.

Another thing that worked for me was to keep looking at pictures of babies, in books, on diaper bags, toilet tissue packages, whatever was handy at the moment. I would do this during a contraction and focus on how all this work was going to bring my baby to me.

At one point, my midwife examined me and said that I had dilated to 7½ centimeters. Everyone cheered. Unfortunately, she added, the lip of the cervix had caught on the baby's head. She reached in to slip it back and that hurt so much they nearly had to pry me off the ceiling. But then, I was over 8 centimeters dilated.

Throughout this process, I couldn't sleep, even after everyone else, except my best friend, had passed out on couches, chairs, the floor. My friend held my hand as I lay on the bed, too tired to move. The waves of pain just kept coming, and I preferred to be awake and ready for them rather than jolted awake in the crest of one.

Until then I had no idea how much physical pain the human body can endure and still survive: I began to feel that I'd had life way too easy.

One friend had brought her two-year-old daughter over, and at one point the child asked, "Mommy, why is that lady screaming?" As soon as the contraction had ended, I said to her, "See, it hurts for just a little while, and then you get a baby." (Years later, this little girl became my son's "big sister." When he started school, she excitedly told her friends, "I watched him being born.")

Finally, the next morning, the midwife broke my water with her fingernail (wearing her rubber gloves, of course). She had warned me that the friction from the baby's hair would increase the sensation of pain, but she said it would also quicken the birth process. Well, it did. I felt like I'd found myself on a tricycle, on a busy freeway trying to keep up with the traffic.

After the midwife broke my water, it took only a few contractions for the widest part of the baby's head to emerge from the cervix, and at last I could push. The midwife gave me a hand mirror so I could see what was happening. She put warm compresses on my perineum to help it stretch and to prevent tearing. I squatted, I stood, I lay on my side, I got on all fours. Somehow the contractions seemed less painful once I could do something with them. But then the midwife wanted me *not* to push for a few contractions. That's when the breathing exercises came in handy, to help me slow down the pushing and avoid tearing. I remember my emotions more clearly than what I felt physically at that point: I was exhausted, excited, and impatient to see who my child would be.

My midwife was squatting behind me. I was crouching, clutching a stool for balance, and looking in the hand mirror. I could see what looked like a very pointy, purplish tip of the baby's head coming out of me; it was a frightening moment. I asked, "Why is the head so small?" My midwife replied, "It's okay; the head is made to do that. It goes back into shape afterward. That's what the fontanelles are for." Then, I was afraid I might have a bowel movement. I told the midwife, and she said, "Don't worry, I'm used to it. I catch a lot of sh__ in my profession."

The baby's head crowned, and then the rest of the baby slipped out easily. It was the most awe-inspiring sensation, feeling my child slide out of me, recognizing the feel of a shoulder, an arm, the hips. This whole person no one had ever met or seen before had just slipped out of me! It was May 11, 1994, 11:30 a.m.

As the midwife caught my son, Jesse, and wiped off his face, my exhausted coaches started to cheer and clap. The midwife quieted them, explaining that the baby might be afraid of all that noise. After all, we were strangers to him, too.

Moments later, as he lay on my stomach, looking placidly up at me and the circle of smiling faces around us, the midwife held the umbilical cord, waiting for it to close itself off before cutting it. Despite smears of vernix, and blood, Jesse was beautiful, with huge wide-open blue eyes that seemed to take in everything around him. I barely even noticed the contractions that pushed out the placenta. By then, he'd begun nursing with gusto. His round, wet head was exactly the size of my breast. He looked up at me as if to say, "So this is how it all works."

The midwife examined my placenta and showed me the spot where it had torn. There was a long scar on the tissue. Then she measured and weighed Jesse. He was 8 pounds, 6 ounces and 21 inches long.

Over the next few days, I lay in bed as much as possible. Jesse lay beside me, nursing whenever he felt like it. I slept when he did (which was a lot). One by one, I peeled off all the layers of sheets my friend so thoughtfully set up, and felt grateful to her every time I did so. Friends and family came by with food and baby gifts. The midwife returned a few days later for our first postnatal checkup. Jesse and I were both in great health. But I have to say, my experience with labor and birth utterly changed my definition of "unbearable pain"!

A Pushless Delivery

*Cathy and David were both 32 years old when their first
child was born in a Los Angeles hospital. At the time, Cathy
was a third-year law student. Because of a serious eye condition,
she was advised to avoid the pushing stage of birth. To do so,
Cathy was scheduled to receive an early epidural and told
to expect forceps or vacuum assistance to achieve a no-push
delivery. Here David, who works in marketing communications,
tells their birth story. "These are the facts of Sonia's birth,"
he writes. "Don't believe Cathy if she disputes them. By her
own admission, she was under the influence of a controlled
substance at the time, and can't be trusted."*

C athy gave birth to our first child, Sonia Elizabeth Marie, on
February 13 in Los Angeles.

We had arrived at the hospital at about 4:30 p.m. on February 12 and proceeded directly to Labor and Delivery, where we were assigned a labor room. Cathy donned the simple yet stylish hospital gown, provided a urine sample, and had her cervical exam. The OB resident pronounced her 3 to 4 centimeters dilated.

This was good news. It meant that the miraculous process of birth was well under way. It meant that we would soon be blessed by the arrival of our first child. It meant that we would not be sent home in shame and humiliation for having gone to the hospital too early.

But, having spared us this cataclysmic loss of face, the resident couldn't resist an insulting innuendo. "First labors are notoriously slow to progress," she said; we should walk around for a couple of hours to help speed things up.

Well, who did she think she was dealing with? A couple of high-strung gun-jumpers who raced to the hospital with the first contraction and stood at the door whimpering to be let in like a pair of poodles? A couple of nervous Nellies? We'd show her a thing or two. Why, we'd "walk around for a couple of hours" and return to the hospital having delivered the child ourselves between dance numbers at some tony nightclub!

As Cathy began changing back into her own clothes, the resident mentioned that she could simply remain in her gown while walking around the hospital. "The hospital?" we thought. "This hospital isn't big enough to hold a couple of free spirits like us. We plan to walk around the neighborhood for starters."

So at about 5:00 p.m., we strode bravely from the comfort of our medical sanctuary and into the exhilarating uncertainty under the open sky.

Moments after stepping from the hospital to the parking structure, Cathy's purposeful gait faltered and we stopped. She said that she was feeling something, something different, something wet. Retreating to a nearby restroom, she discovered that she was wet, but not wet enough that she could be certain her water had broken. After a brief conference ("What do you think?" "I don't know. What do you think?" "I don't know, what do you think?"), we decided to press ahead with our walk.

We set out for my nearby office building to pick up my workout bag (the idea being that I would experience a burst of paternal vigor at some point during the weekend and would need to exercise).

Our progress was slow. With each contraction—and the contractions were coming far more frequently now that we were on the move—we would pause in our journey. Cathy would do breathing exercises to help her control the pain while I would hold her in my arms and murmur words of soothing reassurance: "Relax," "You're doing great," "I love you," and "Don't spew our child onto the dirt."

Slowly and unsteadily, we made it to my office. Cathy visited the restroom again and we held another conference ("I don't know. What do you think?"). As we were setting no land-speed records, we decided to start our return trip immediately. Once under way, we decided that it would be prudent for us to have a quick taco.

Then, we made our slow and unsteady way back to the hospital with plenty of pausing, breathing, and murmuring. After a final restroom stop near the hospital's entrance and a final conference ("I think so. Don't you think so?"), we returned to Labor and Delivery at about 7:00 p.m.

Cathy was examined again, and yes, her water had indeed broken. We were told that she wouldn't be walking anywhere again that evening.

Because of an eye condition Cathy has, she had been advised by her ophthalmologist that the extreme stress of pushing a baby out could cause her to damage or even lose her sight. For that reason it was decided in advance that she would have an early-stage epidural and a no-pushing delivery. So the next order of business was to begin giving her some drugs. After the anesthesiologist explained the possible risks of the anesthesia, the labor nurse attempted to start an IV. Too bad the anesthesiologist hadn't seen fit to explain the risks of starting an IV. If he had, Cathy might have been prepared for all the bruises. On the fourth attempt (two by the nurse, two by the doctor), they finally managed to place the IV.

With this accomplished, the anesthesiologist asked me to step out of the room for a few minutes while he placed the epidural in Cathy's spine. After the episode with the IV, it was clear to me that he intended to botch this next procedure so cruelly that he didn't dare allow me to witness the debacle.

When I returned a short time later, I was surprised to discover a smiling and carefree young woman sitting in my wife's bed chatting happily with the labor nurse. I was even more surprised to discover that the smiling young woman was my wife.

From this point on, Cathy's labor progressed smoothly and steadily. Her body continued its work of preparing to expel this child that had been growing there since the previous May. At about 11:30 p.m., the OB resident examined Cathy again and announced that she was 10 centimeters dilated . . . it was *showtime*!

They wheeled her from her labor room, which had been like the small extra bedroom in the house of someone with bad taste, to the delivery room, a very large and well-lit medical-looking place with that scary professional decor. Our labor nurse built a nest of disposable paper and plastic items around Cathy's lower half and laid out a collection of doctors' tools that reminded me of an extravagant place setting at some fancy dinner party where you don't know what half the utensils are to be used for. The collection included a couple of distressingly large sets of forceps—I mean really giant ones that would dwarf your average set of salad tongs.

As the nurse completed her preparations, Cathy's obstetrician and the OB resident who had examined Cathy throughout the evening came in and squirmed into their surgical gowns. (Use of the hands is considered cheating and is frowned upon.) The OB resident was difficult to recognize because, in addition to her surgical mask, she wore racquetball eye protectors. Yikes! Was it going to be that messy?!

While a good batch of modern chemistry's finest was keeping Cathy comfortable, she would be left to labor the baby down into the canal as far as possible without pushing. The OB would rely on Cathy's uterine contractions alone to move the baby to a point where she could use forceps or suction to help pull the baby the rest of the way out.

When the doctor examined Cathy in the delivery room, she was pleasantly surprised to see that her contractions had pushed the baby nearly to the point of delivery. Who wouldn't be pleased with a paying customer who did most of the work herself?

The only hitch was that the baby was "sunny side up," the opposite of most babies, who leave the uterus facing the mother's spine. Using a

184

single blade of the forceps, the doctors tried twice to turn the baby like a bird on a rotisserie. Both times, the baby promptly turned back to its preferred orientation.

To assist in the birth, the doctors then attached a suction cup to the baby's head and prepared to pull it out with the next contraction. The baby picked that moment to rotate all on its own into the normal, face-down position. Who needs doctors, anyway?

The next contraction came and the OB resident pulled on the suction cup. Now, don't get the idea that this was some delicate medical procedure requiring a steady hand and a gentle touch. It more closely resembled a tug-of-war between the OB resident and some powerful and stubborn creature that had taken refuge between Cathy's thighs. The pressure increased and the tension mounted until, with a tremendous *pop*, the suction cup came unstuck from the baby's head. The OB and the OB resident quickly reat-

I CAN'T OVER-STATE HOW STRANGE IT WAS TO SEE A BABY'S HEAD FIRMLY WEDGED BETWEEN MY WIFE'S LEGS.

tached it and the contest began anew. Now the pulling grew really fierce. I would have become concerned if my auto mechanic were to apply such force in removing a part from our Jeep.

The OB began chanting, "Here it comes, here it comes," to reassure the parents and to convince the baby that further resistance would be futile. And then, before my eyes, the baby's head spun into view, face upward.

I can't overstate how strange it was to see a baby's head firmly wedged between my wife's legs.

At this point, the delivery paused briefly to allow the nurse to suction the baby's airways (the mouth and both nostrils) and to await the next contraction to help deliver the baby's shoulders.

But the intermission was very brief and with a steady pull by the OB resident to assist Cathy's contraction, the rest of the baby slid into the open air. As her wrinkled little body flashed by, I caught a glimpse of her swollen genitalia and delivered my only meaningful line in the drama, "It's a girl!"

Cathy had delivered Sonia directly into the doctor's disposably gloved hands. The other disposable items caught the rest of the mushy puddle and were promptly thrown away. Things were tidy again in no time.

Quick and Easy

*Denise, a counselor in a local mental health center,
was 29 when her first child was born
in a hospital in North Carolina. Her husband, Bob, was 40 and
working as a controller for a furniture manufacturer. These are the
entries for the last few days of her pregnancy journal.*

Wednesday, October 16

My energy level has dropped precipitously the past week. Work, home, wherever. Zero pep. At least I slept well last night; didn't wake up once. Little Bit's getting the hiccups at least once or twice a day now. And still kicking like the dickens. One month to go, give or take 14 days.

Saturday, October 19

Everyone says I'm looking real good. I'm thankful this pregnancy is going so smoothly. I'll take a puffy ankle or two and a little back soreness compared to some of the things folks I know had to go through. I just hope my good luck carries through the labor and delivery. I'm afraid something will go wrong and hurt the baby. I'm afraid of pain. I'm afraid.

Tuesday, October 29

Went for a checkup. Everything is fine. I told the doctor I felt the baby turn out of the breech position a few days ago. He told me there was no way I could possibly know that. Then he palpated my abdomen and announced, with surprise, that I was right!

Wednesday, October 30

The folks at the office gave me a baby shower today—lots of goodies for Little Bit. It was a pretty good day, but I started to feel a little punky about midafternoon. The fireplace doors came back; they fit perfectly and look wonderful.

The Braxton Hicks contractions are coming stronger and more frequently. Bit's also kicking stronger. The baby is so big now, I feel stuffed.

Thursday, October 31

Worn out. Wasn't really hungry, just ate a pot pie for dinner. Went up to bed at 8:30.

Friday, November 1 [Written three days later, the day after coming home from the hospital]

Surprise, surprise! Guess who showed up two weeks early?

I had the most atypical labor pattern I've ever heard of. I woke up at 1:00 a.m. needing to pee, normal for the past several weeks. No sooner had I returned to bed than I needed to pee again; in fact, I thought I had wet my pants rushing to the bathroom and was both embarrassed and annoyed. (I later discovered that had been my water breaking and that the baby had dropped so low that her head was damming the flow to a trickle.) This pattern continued for the next five and a half hours, except I added diarrhea from about 3:00 a.m., plus nausea and vomiting, and regular contractions (about every 10 minutes) from about 4:00 a.m. on.

This whole time, I had no inkling I might be in real labor. I only became concerned when I noticed I'd been passing blood. At around 6:30 a.m., I called the doctor's office and got a recording with no paging number, so I called the hospital. The nurse told me to come on in and they'd check me out, but neither my husband, Bob, nor I thought it was urgent at that point.

Bob took a quick shower while I put on some clothes. He had to put my shoes on for me. At that point, the contractions kicked in about every three minutes and they felt like a hard squeezing. But I still didn't think it was real, active labor because they didn't really hurt, though they were strong enough to interfere with my ability to walk.

In the car, the contractions became stronger and I had to start using my breathing techniques. They still didn't feel that painful. The main problem was I couldn't breathe normally during them. Once we got on Highway 90, Bob decided that this was probably the one time we could speed and not get a ticket. So, he jammed the accelerator, hazard lights and high beams flashing. Politely, every car pulled over for us. I did my breathing exercises and kept my eyes closed. Bob told me he was going 75 miles per hour; he later admitted he was really doing 90. We made it to the hospital (normally a 20- to 25-minute trip) in 12 minutes flat.

I walked into the hospital, but by the time they asked if I wanted to walk up to my floor or go in a wheelchair, I couldn't walk anymore. They wheeled me up to a Labor and Delivery room, helped me undress and put on a gown, then did the preliminary exam. I was 8 centimeters dilated already and the baby was at zero station, its head in my pelvis, so they called the doctor immediately. My contractions, which had been two minutes apart, increased in frequency and got stronger. Now they felt like giant hands wrapped around my abdomen, squeezing down. I wanted to push, but the nurses wouldn't let me push until the doctor got there, so I yelled instead. They tried to put me on the fetal monitor, but never could get it placed right to monitor the contractions. However, they did find out that the baby's heart rate had dropped a bit, so they put me on oxygen. Bob tried to take off my glasses, but I told him not to because I wanted to see (although I'm pretty sure I kept my eyes closed most of the time).

Finally, I reached the point where I couldn't *not* push, and just as I was about to tell them I didn't care if a candy striper delivered my baby, I heard the magic words, "The doctor's here." He yelled into the room and asked if he had time to change into surgical scrubs. They all said, "No!" so in he came wearing jeans and tassel loafers. The nurse helped him slip on paper booties, a paper bonnet, a gown, and gloves, and he sat down. (Bob told me afterward that for some reason he noticed that the tassel of one shoe had gotten caught outside the bootie.) Finally, they let me sit up and push. I wanted to sit completely upright and push down, again feeling those giant hands pushing through me. You've heard Carol Burnett's joke about pushing a watermelon through an opening the size of an orange? Well, it's accurate. But painful as it was, I never had any sense that I couldn't do it or that my body wasn't doing what it needed to do. It was unnerving in that it was involuntary, but at the same time, I had a strong sense that my body was doing something that had happened billions of times before, and it knew what to do. All I needed to do was stay out of the way and keep calm. It was in many ways an intensely spiritual experience.

Then I felt the head coming out. This is the only part that I remember as being truly painful. I thought I could feel the head moving down, but people had told me that you usually think it's moving down when it's not, so I still didn't believe this thing was happening so quickly. Then suddenly the pain stopped, as if someone had turned off a switch. The head was out. They suctioned it, then I asked if I could push again. The doctor kind of laughed and said there wasn't any need, but I felt I needed to, so I did. The

I HAD A STRONG SENSE THAT MY BODY WAS DOING SOMETHING THAT HAD HAPPENED BILLIONS OF TIMES BEFORE, AND IT KNEW WHAT TO DO.

rest of the body was born almost immediately, and then we saw we had a healthy baby girl. Dorothea Elizabeth weighed in at 6 pounds, 8 ounces and was 19 inches long. She was nursing within five minutes, right there on the delivery table. She was born at 7:48 a.m.; we'd checked into the hospital at 7:20.

They took her to the nursery for all her tests, and I cleaned up a little while Bob made some phone calls. I called work at 8:30 a.m. to say I wouldn't be in, then they brought breakfast for me and Bob. At 9:20, I was moved to my postpartum room and Thea was brought in soon after.

She was incredible. Perfect! Ten fingers, ten toes, not even too misshapen from molding through the pelvis. Swathed in a blanket with a little stocking cap on her head, she lay on her side with her eyes open, just looking around. I fed her a couple of times the first day and changed her first diaper. She doesn't look like either Bob or me. But she feels like mine.

2:00 p.m.

Mom and Dad arrive, followed by Grandma and Grandpa D. We didn't know they were coming. Bob had forgotten to tell Mom and Dad the baby's name when he called them on the phone, so we got to tell Grandma face-to-face that we'd named our daughter after her, and she started crying. Everybody had to hold Thea and take pictures; she was an angel through it all—didn't cry once (until she got hungry). Bob said Dad got all teary-eyed down in the lobby.

They all stayed until about 5:00 p.m., then headed home. Later Bob came back for one more visit. Then I was alone with my baby girl. The reality of this took some getting used to. Thea was only content when held, so at 4:00 a.m. the nurse took her so I could get some sleep.

After Exhaustion and Agony, Joy

Irene, a German woman, had her first child at the age of 40 in hospital in Hamburg. She was a sales representative for a large corporation before her son's birth. Her husband, Harald, was 42, and worked as an insurance agent.

I was in my 40th week, so when I woke up at 1:30 a.m. from a slight twinge in my abdomen, I immediately knew this was going to be the day. I was too excited to go back to sleep, so I got up, silently, not wanting to alarm my husband too early. I walked around the living room waiting for the next twinge, which came about 20 minutes later. At 2:30 a.m. I took a bath as my midwife had told me to do, to make sure I would not be fooled by false contractions. Lying in the bathtub, I talked to my baby, telling him that this would probably be a hard day for both of us, but that together we would work it out.

After the bath, the contractions came a bit heavier and they were already every 10 minutes, so I decided to wake up my husband. He was so excited, he jumped right out of bed and didn't know what to do first. When I had calmed him down, I called the hospital to let them know we would be coming soon.

At 4:30 a.m. I was admitted to the hospital. By that time, my labor pains were already quite heavy. A midwife led us into a room where she examined me and plugged me into the monitor. The contractions were coming every five minutes. My midwife told me how to breathe and told me to say "yes" to every contraction because that would help to let my baby come out. That was easier said than done.

Around 7:00, I went into my room and had some breakfast. At that time I was still able to breathe through the pain. At 9:00 a.m., they brought me to the delivery room for another examination and again hooked me up to the monitor.

The next two hours were very tough. Contractions were coming one after the other, each lasting perhaps one minute. I did not expect it to be that painful. It was like somebody was working on me with a knife. I could not lie on the bed anymore, so I used the "Pezzi" ball, which offered some relief. (The Pezzi ball is a large rubber ball, about two feet high, which you sit on. If you straddle it, with your legs wide open, it relieves the pressure on the pelvis and eases the pain.) The midwife suggested that I take a bath, but I refused. I had no desire to stand up and move to the bathtub. By now my husband was crying, as he couldn't bear to see me in such pain.

Around 11:00 a.m., I asked for pain relief, and they gave me an injection. It did relieve the pain, but unfortunately, my contractions stopped. I was told to walk around in order to stabilize my blood circulation, but suddenly the baby had a problem, so I was on the bed again. They gave me some oxygen and the baby was okay, but now they wanted to monitor me, so I stayed in the delivery room.

At 2:00 p.m. the doctor in charge decided to get my labor back into progress with the help of Pitocin, given intravenously. As they expected this to be very painful for a couple of hours and didn't think I could bear it, they also suggested an epidural.

A while later, the anesthesiologist came and told my husband to go have some lunch. By the time he'd finished his work and switched on the infusion, it was 3:00.

I was very curious about what would happen next, and afraid of more pain, but I also wanted my baby. The contractions started out quite heavy, as I could see by looking at the monitor, but because of the epidural, I felt nothing. The next two hours were quite relaxing. I talked and joked with my husband and the midwife, who checked on me every half-hour to see if my cervix was opening wider. This was the third midwife who had cared for me since I had arrived at the hospital.

BECAUSE OF THE EPIDURAL, I FELT NOTHING. THE NEXT TWO HOURS WERE QUITE RELAXING. I TALKED AND JOKED WITH MY HUSBAND AND THE MIDWIFE.

At 5:00 p.m., my cervix was fully dilated. The midwife burst my bag of water and expected the baby to come soon, but nothing happened. As the epidural began to wear off, I could feel the contractions again, and I didn't know how to lie quietly anymore. At 6:00 they gave me more anesthetic through the drip tube, and the pain lessened but did not vanish completely. The next three hours were extremely strenuous. I didn't feel the contractions much, but the baby was causing pain by pushing against parts of me that were unaffected by the anesthesia—especially my stomach. I was tired, impatient, and in pain, my husband was exhausted, and the baby seemed to like it just where he was. It seemed that he simply was not going to move deep enough into the birth canal.

At 9:00 p.m., they decided to give me one more shot of anesthetic. I fell asleep for an hour. When I woke up, I told the doctor that I didn't want to wait any longer, I wanted her to get the baby out—now! As the baby seemed to be exhausted, too, and the pain was getting worse every minute, they decided to get the baby out by means of vacuum suction.

The next hour I went through hell. All I remember is that my husband had to press the oxygen mask on my face because the baby's heart rate was getting lower and lower, and that I wanted to go home. After the second push, I told them to stop, I had had enough, I could not bear it any longer. But it is amazing what you can bear. It took 30 minutes for three birth contractions. Each time, I pushed for about one minute while one doctor used the vacuum and a second doctor pressed into my belly with his whole weight. They encouraged me to push once more. The baby was almost out, he only needed one more push, so I pressed and pressed and pressed and finally, I felt him coming out. He was born at 11:05 p.m.

I just can't describe the feelings I had when they put the baby on my body. It was overwhelming. My husband and I were crying for joy. It was the happiest moment of my life. I held Robert in my arms and I just couldn't believe how cute he was, my precious little baby.

After a few minutes, one of the doctors and my husband took the baby away from me to check him. I was quite relieved they did because I now felt extremely exhausted. I was still plugged in to the intravenous setup and could feel the afterbirth contractions quite heavily. The anesthesia was completely gone by now. The midwife delivered the placenta and then washed and dressed me. I had to stay on the same bed until they could move me onto a clean one. Because I had been on anesthesia for eight hours, my blood pressure was very low and they kept me under observation in the delivery room for an hour and a half.

While the midwife was stitching my episiotomy, my husband and the doctor were taking care of the baby. He passed the Apgar tests and they washed and dressed him. When I saw Harald sitting on a chair, holding a little white parcel on his lap, I just couldn't believe that he was holding our son. I felt very proud, also, for my husband who had suffered with me and stood by me the whole long day.

After I was cleaned and moved to the new bed, I was given the baby for a while. The midwife helped me put him to my breast. He sucked for a while, but I'm not sure if anything came out. Then Harald, Robert, and I relaxed. Around 1:00 a.m., they took the baby to the nursery. (Hospital policy is to monitor babies the first night.) My husband went home and I was sent to bed, but I was still too excited to sleep. Luckily I had a roommate who was willing to talk with me about this extraordinary experience.

At 5:00 a.m. they brought my baby back. From that moment on, he was all mine.

The Water
Took It All

*Debbie writes, "I was 36 and my husband, Ivan,
was 58 when our son was born at home, in the Bronx,
New York. Because we publish an educational resource guide,*
The Book of TLC, *on health and disease, I've reviewed
thousands of audio and video titles. When I saw my
first water birth on video, I knew that was for me."*

M y due date was the first week of November. On November 2, I had fallen asleep at 9:00 p.m. About a half hour later, I was awakened by the feeling of water on my legs and I thought I had wet my pants. It wasn't much fluid. I was still very drowsy, so I went right back to sleep. A few minutes later, my mother called, waking me up, and I told her about the fluid. My mother, who had six children, said, "Well, your water probably broke. Why don't you call your midwife and let her know?" My midwife, who was very laissez-faire, said, "Well, okay, go back to bed. We probably have another twenty-four hours, maybe longer. Relax. It's just the beginning." Relax? How could I? I was excited. This was it.

But I finally went back to sleep, feeling little contractions throughout the night, like tiny cramps hugging my uterus, every 15 minutes. They didn't hurt, but I knew my body was getting ready for the bigger contractions. For the past few weeks, my doula and I had been practicing meditation to help me visualize the labor and birth. I usually visualized my baby coming down a water slide. I also thought a lot about my body preparing itself for the journey to the birth.

The next morning I woke up feeling great. I was still having contractions. I called the people who were to be with me at the birth: my girlfriend Michelle, who was going to assist me and document the birth by taking photographs and video, and my doula, Judith, who specialized in water births. Ivan, my husband, was already home with me. I remember looking out the window at 11:30 a.m., waving to friends walking by and calling out, "Hey, I'm in labor!"

I spent a lot of time walking around the apartment. Often, I would stop in the smooth archway between two rooms and press my back against one side of the arch, while doing leg lunges against the other side. The lunges helped relieve the pain in my lower back. I didn't feel the hugging of the contractions anymore. All the pressure was now on my back. The contractions were getting stronger, closer, about eight minutes apart, lasting 30 to 60 seconds. Eventually, they lasted 90 seconds.

During this early labor, I also sat on an inflated exercise ball, about three feet in diameter, and rocked on it, to keep my hips loose. It was a good distraction for me. I also watched a video called *Down Below*, which showed underwater scenes of sea life, accompanied by New Age music. It was very relaxing.

Meanwhile, Ivan and I tried to figure out when to set up the birthing tub provided by our doula. She rents it to people for five weeks at a time so they will be sure to have it in the house when labor begins. It's five feet in diameter, with sides about three or four feet high, and made of vinyl. It looks like an oversized, colorful kiddie pool, complete with a graphic of the New York City skyline. We decided to wait until Michelle arrived, so she could help. She got there at about 1:00 p.m. Unfortunately, she and Ivan had some trouble. The water was too hot, and it was coming out of the pipes all brown. With water that color, I couldn't even fill our regular bathtub and use it for labor.

I called my midwife and told her my contractions were getting stronger. She had attended a birth that morning, and told me she had a post-delivery checkup scheduled for that afternoon. After the checkup, she planned to drive back to her home in Brooklyn to pick up clean instruments and then drive to the Bronx. For months, my mother had reminded me about her very short labors, but the midwife and I weren't really taking that into account.

Judith, my doula, arrived about 3:30 p.m. and made me a special pot of labor tea with raspberry leaf, nettles, blessed thistle, fennel, and honey. (It was a huge pot of tea—when she asked my husband for a pot, he gave her a stew pot!) We called my midwife again, and I told her everything felt essentially the same as before; things were changing, but only gradually. About 15 minutes after hanging up the phone though, my contractions became more intense and started coming every couple of minutes, really one on top of another. I felt like I couldn't catch my breath between them. Judith was applying counter-pressure on my back, where I felt the contractions most, which was very helpful. Ivan and Michelle were still working with the tub and preparing the bed, layering it with sheets and plastic and towels.

At 3:45 p.m. my hardest labor began. I vomited twice, but we had been prepared for this possibility, with a bucket ready in the bedroom. By now I was having a hard time finding a comfortable position. The hormones were affecting my legs, which were shaking, but I didn't want to lie down. I was still pacing around and trying to straddle a chair cushioned by a pillow. My doula kept whispering in my ear, "Trust your body, your body knows how to birth; you're doing a fantastic job," and, "Trust your baby; your baby knows how."

About 4:45, Ivan phoned my midwife again. Judith, who was at my side, told him to say that I was now in active labor. My midwife was on her way to Brooklyn to pick up her clean instruments and would then come directly to us.

At about 5:00 p.m. the tub was finally ready. I tried getting into the water a few times, but it wasn't deep enough and I really wasn't comfortable there. Lying down at this point was impossible. I was more comfortable being vertical, straddling a chair, leaning over it with a pillow. I did this until around 6:00. We were playing the soundtrack from the movie *The Piano*, some very penetrating piano music. It's funny: I don't remember much about this time period—I was concentrating so hard on what was going on in my body—but to this day, I have very intense feelings when I hear that music.

Sometime before 7:00 p.m., I got back into the water and then got out again. My midwife called from her car and said she was on the way, but now she was stuck in traffic. I knew she wasn't going to get there in time, but I wasn't worried. I felt secure, being with people who loved me and whom I trusted.

All of a sudden, right after the phone call from my midwife, I felt all this pressure in my rectum. So I said to Judith, "I feel so much pressure, I think I need to push." Judith said, "Well, then, you probably need to push. Let's get back into the tub."

> **MY DOULA KEPT WHISPERING IN MY EAR, "TRUST YOUR BODY, YOUR BODY KNOWS HOW TO BIRTH; YOU'RE DOING A FANTASTIC JOB," AND, "TRUST YOUR BABY; YOUR BABY KNOWS HOW."**

Judith and my husband got in the tub with me. At this point, Judith wanted to check me internally, my first internal exam since my labor began. She stuck her fingers gently inside me, and felt the baby's head. It was soft and surrounded by fluid. We realized then that the baby was still in his sac. Judith and Ivan talked about our options. By now I couldn't speak. I just made sure I heard what they were saying.

I was absorbed by my task, and I wasn't the least bit worried. The room was filled with candlelight and soft music. Everything was very serene. Our child had already chosen his own name: Sage. Ivan said he could feel Sage's spirit all around, and Sage said, "Let nature take its course. Let the water break by itself." Meanwhile, Michelle was quietly documenting the birth on video.

I was in a kind of kneeling squat, on all fours, leaning forward against the pool's side so that my butt was down in the water, angled, creating that water slide I had visualized, though I wasn't aware of it at the time. Beforehand, I had thought I would simply be squatting, but my legs were so tired, I decided kneeling would be better. My husband was still in the tub, stroking my back, and Judith, my doula, was sitting in the water behind me. I was in a pretty good mood most of the time. I only snapped at them once, to ask them to turn down the music because it was bothering me. At this point, I wanted my husband to stroke my back. That felt great.

We tried to keep the tub water at about 95 degrees and we turned the thermostat up in our apartment. The water was only about two and a half feet deep—not deep enough for me to float or feel buoyant, but it was very relaxing. Being in the water made it much easier for me first to imagine my muscles opening and then to open them. I had taken only baths my whole pregnancy, no showers, so I felt very comforted and soothed.

It also helped that Ivan was very tuned in to my needs the whole time. He knew what I needed without asking. Sometimes he was there with me; other times he was preparing things for me. He knew how to weave himself in and out of the intense feminine energy he was surrounded by. Maybe our childbirth classes had helped. We had taken two private classes, one on water births, and one dealing with pain management. In the pain management class, Ivan was asked to squat and lean against a wall for a long time to get an idea of what I might be going through in labor—how my legs might cramp, how my back might feel. And I had to figure out exactly how I would deal with the pain, so that Ivan would be able to recognize what I was experiencing and be able to help me.

The contractions had slowed a little once I got into the water. (For this reason, it is recommended that you do not get into the water before you are dilated 5 centimeters. I didn't know how far I was dilated. I just knew being in the water didn't feel right in the early stages.) Judith, still behind me, was trying to help me keep my butt in the water.

My sounds changed now, becoming very deep and guttural, animalistic. Earlier, the noises I'd made had been higher-pitched, more sensual. In between contractions, I was saying to my son, "Come on. Come out. You can do it." In about two pushes, perhaps eight minutes apart, he crowned. With the next contraction, I pushed his head, shoulders, and arms out. I could feel it was his head, but I felt no "ring of fire," no pain. I think the water took it all away.

Afterward, looking at the video, I could see that when his head came out, he was still veiled by his amniotic sac. It was floating in the water, to his side. It reminded me of the sea plankton I'd seen earlier on the underwater film.

Ivan was in front of me, still stroking my back, talking to me, vocalizing with me, with my loud, deep grunts. Judith was still behind me, in the water. She was telling me, "Come on, just a couple more pushes." Michelle and Judith could see the baby, and they were both saying, "Oh, he's so beautiful!"

It seemed that time stopped for me here. Judith calls this period, "Restitution," when the baby is half-in, half-out, gathering strength to come all the way out. She asked me, "Debbie, do you want to push?"

And I said, "No, not really. I want to wait." I could barely hear her. I was just waiting for the contraction to tell me when to push.

Then it came. My next push. For the first time in the entire labor, I could feel the whole baby in my front. My whole abdomen and stomach just pushed the baby out, like a huge sigh of relief. And I said to myself, "I did it!" This last push didn't even hurt.

Sometime after he came out, I don't know when exactly, the veil detached and was left in the water. When the baby was completely out, Judith took him and slid him between my legs, underwater, and brought him up toward my husband who very sweetly wanted me to have the honor of holding him first, but I couldn't. I was too tired. I just wanted to recoup my energy for a moment. So Ivan picked him up out of the water and said, "Welcome, Sweet Pea."

Sage's eyes were open and he was looking at us, very aware. Judith rubbed his back and his feet, waiting for him to take a breath. She was a bit worried because he wasn't breathing yet, but I was confident that he was all right. I said, "He'll be fine." I knew I was blessed. My intense feelings of love and trust seemed to leave no room for fear or doubt. Judith was holding Sage now, and she blew into his nose, very gently, a technique she'd learned only two weeks earlier at a workshop. He cried out, and then he breathed.

I sat down in the water, spread my legs to relax them, held my baby, and congratulated myself. I fully realized the impact of the moment only then. My husband phoned my mother. My midwife was at the door, and perhaps she had been for a few minutes, but we hadn't heard the doorbell until that moment. She came in, and we all said, "We did it!"

She immediately checked the cord, took a blood sample from it, and got it ready for Ivan to cut it. Then Ivan cut the cord. I was leaning back against the cushion of the tub, still sitting with my legs spread out. My midwife rubbed my belly a bit, pulled on the cord a little and the placenta popped out, with no contraction.

I sat in the tub for about half an hour, holding the baby. I tried to nurse him, but he wasn't interested. I was just relaxing. The water was bloody, but it didn't bother me. I was too amazed by everything. The baby was so aware, looking all around, taking everything in. It was all very peaceful. Then, Ivan took him, and I got out of the tub.

As I got out of the tub, I felt a little stinging, and when I told the midwife, she said, "Well, you probably tore." I needed 10 stitches, for a second-degree tear. For me, this was the worst part of the birth. I had a little anesthesia and lay on my side on the bed as she stitched me. Judith lay next to me, talking and distracting me from the stitching. It didn't hurt, exactly. I just didn't like it.

Everyone left at about 1:00 a.m. I could hardly sleep the first night; Sage slept on my belly and I alternately dozed and gazed at my beautiful baby.

My husband and I had been together 15 years, and I was 36 years old. I had waited to become pregnant because I wanted to be emotionally ready for being a parent. Sage's birth marked a real transition for me: from a woman to a mother. His birth heightened my awareness of my own physicality and the genius of our bodies. For the first time, I felt really connected to creation. And I felt empowered.

Lessons for Life

*Lani was married and a 28-year-old actress when her
son was delivered by a midwife in a Manhattan hospital
in 1988. Seven years later, when her daughter came
along, she was single and a graduate student.*

My first experience with labor was in 1988, when Zachary
was born. That night, I was supposed to go to a party, but
by early evening, I was feeling achy and queasy in my
stomach and called to say I was coming down with "some stomach
thing" and was staying home. It never occurred to me that I was
actually going into labor. Zach was due only four days later, on January 7, but my symptoms weren't very dramatic, so I didn't make the
connection.

Eight hours later, around midnight, it was clear I was in labor. I was
having spasms of stomach pressure at regular intervals, about every 15
minutes, sometimes even 10 minutes. I spoke to Maureen, my midwife, a
few times after midnight, and she kept track of what seemed to be very
early and insignificant labor. By 4:00 a.m., however, I had a feeling I
should go to the hospital, even though the contractions didn't seem all

that severe. Maureen agreed with me because she's kind and accommo-
dating, not because it seemed to her that anything much was happening.

I headed out the door on January 3, 1988 with my then-husband to
hail a taxi. We went crashing through the potholes of Times Square
while I tried to keep myself off the seat by hanging from a handle in the
cab. From the moment I left home, I had been plunging into squats at
every contraction as I walked along the sidewalk in my full-length win-
ter coat. This didn't faze me. In fact, I continued to feel unapologetic as
I sank to the floor with each contraction throughout the admission
process at the hospital. I remember this lack of self-consciousness because for me, not being at all concerned with the reactions of others was
a first. I have found since then that motherhood has consistently af-
forded me this kind of freedom.

When Maureen arrived at the hospital and hooked me up to the
monitor, she exclaimed, "You didn't tell me you were in active labor!"
My water hadn't broken and I didn't know what anything was supposed
to feel like, so I was clueless about how far along I was, but glad to hear
I was well on the way. (My water never did break on its own; Maureen
punctured the sac near the end.) Years later, I realized that it was my
tendency to always minimize what happened to me or how I felt. So I
minimized the intensity of what I was feeling and had conveyed very
little of it to Maureen. It's that old "I-can-handle-this" thing.

The hardest and shortest part of labor, I was told in my prenatal
class, is called "transition," the shift from the completion of dilation
to pushing. As it happened, I got stuck in the transition stage, but
Maureen is brilliant and did not see any point in mentioning this, so

I didn't know how "bad" that was. I was given an IV to help with dehydration and later Pitocin to get things going again. While the Pitocin did make things move faster, the rhythm of the contractions was much more jagged for me than my natural labor had been. The contractions were now more stressful, and I agreed to use a painkiller when it was offered to me. What I didn't know then is that the moment you find the whole thing unbearable, it's almost over. (The same thing happened with my second baby, but that time I didn't take the painkiller because I knew the baby was almost out anyway. My sister, and other women I've talked to, however, highly recommend getting an epidural, which allegedly "kills all pain." My feeling is, it's really up to you.)

For both of my births, the pushing was the hardest part because I was so completely exhausted by then, and it felt as though the birth would never happen: I thought the baby just wouldn't come out. With my first baby, I seriously considered just leaving. Then I envisioned myself walking around outside in that stupid little hospital nightgown with the open back, carting an IV around and still having to deal with an unborn baby. The realization that I would only be taking the problem with me took the appeal right out of that idea. With my second baby, just before Isabel made her appearance, I decided to go deeper into the labor and encourage—well, okay, beg!—my body to let the baby come out. And it worked!

From a purely technical standpoint, the glitches in my two labors and deliveries were identical. Both times my labor ground to a halt as the babies got stuck in transition. This may be because both babies were in the posterior position, which causes the dreaded "back labor," when the contractions are painfully centered in your lower back. I didn't know I was having back labor, so I wasn't worried about it. Zachary had the cord wrapped around his neck twice (not that unusual), while Isabel outdid him, managing to wrap it around herself three times. When Maureen asked me to stop pushing with Isabel, though stopping at that moment is extremely difficult, I knew it was important, so I stopped. With Zachary, however, I just wanted to get the baby OUT, and I didn't stop pushing even when I was told to. The result was Maureen had no chance to turn Zachary, and I tore when his shoulder emerged.

> **MY BREATHING CHANGED ON ITS OWN WITH THE DIFFERENT STAGES OF LABOR, DESPITE MY WORRIES THAT I WOULDN'T REMEMBER WHAT I WAS "SUPPOSED" TO DO.**

Zachary was my first full-term pregnancy. I had lost two babies before him, so I was especially anxious about his birth. In fact, I didn't make a peep the whole time, though I noticed with relief that my breathing changed on its own with the different stages of labor, despite my worries that I wouldn't remember what I was "supposed" to do.

At the time of Zachary's birth, I was married to someone I wasn't very connected to, and, frankly, I wasn't very connected to myself either. Neither of us had any self-confidence. For me, giving birth to my son was the beginning of my active participation in the shaping of my own life. When I was in labor with him, I didn't know what would help me; the "soothing" music I had chosen for the occasion drove me crazy once the vicelike contractions were intense enough to demand my full attention. In fact, I found that most of the suggestions from the prenatal classes (soothing music, familiar objects, and whatever else was supposed to be comforting) were not useful at all.

Seven years later, when Isabel came along, I was divorced, in graduate school, and struggling with another completely unsupportive relationship. Isabel's father, a different man, had decided he really wasn't ready to be in a relationship when I was six months pregnant. However, he did like the idea of being a dad and wouldn't leave me alone for fear I would cut him off from his child. These stressful circumstances made my pregnancy a bizarre paradox of torture and peace: torture, because I didn't have the luxury of feeling thoroughly happy about having this child; and peace, because I was forced to learn to be "in my own corner," regardless of what anyone else might think. This gave me a strength that I think, ideally, every woman becoming a mother needs. I would never recommend going through a pregnancy alone, but the experience did give me the courage to become truer to myself.

The real downside of that experience, was that, probably due to all the emotional turmoil I was suffering, I went into false labor three times in the last month of my pregnancy. However, thanks to my previous experience with labor, I did know when it was really time to go to the hospital. My labor with Isabel was three hours shorter than with Zachary, but after all the pre-labor labor, I felt I deserved a delivery that took only minutes!

While I was pregnant with Isabel, I had made a new friend, Ronda, who went through the last part of the pregnancy and labor with me, and it was lovely to be with two women in the delivery room. I took a tiny pillow with me that another dear friend had made for me years before and used it for moaning and sometimes whimpering on. It was very comforting indeed. This time I knew exactly what would feel best and what I wanted: no music and a lot of squatting! Most surprising and helpful were the long, sustained sounds that I found myself making with each contraction.

I WOULD NEVER RECOMMEND GOING THROUGH A PREGNANCY ALONE, BUT THE EXPERIENCE DID GIVE ME THE COURAGE TO BECOME TRUER TO MYSELF.

Before my labor with Isabel, I had worried that I would forget myself, the baby, or God during the intensity of labor. What I found was that those three realities were all I experienced throughout the labor. It was an astonishing time of prayer and connectedness to myself, my body, my baby, and above all, life itself. Near the end of my labor, I was focused on a spot on the wall just above eye-level in front of me; it was like a hole or tunnel of light that completely held my attention and strengthened me in a truly formidable way. I felt I was in the grasp of Grace.

I remember praying to the part of my body where the baby was lodged as I made my exhausted efforts to push her out. I encouraged my body to blossom into opening, much like a flower, and to let poor little Isabel out. Then Ronda and Maureen pushed my knees up and my head down—as if I were doing a vertical abdominal crunch—and helped me squeeze her out, her eyes open as her head appeared among us.

Both times I thought for all of two days after the birth that I couldn't possibly do that again, but life with those heavenly creatures changed my mind completely within days.

There is no real way of saying what it feels like to give birth, because there is truly nothing that compares. I cannot think of another experience with an outcome so astonishingly and overpoweringly beautiful that it makes such torturous work worth doing.

Thanks to having endured labor and delivery, I can now endure— sometimes even enjoy—some of the most difficult experiences of life. I have thought of labor as a valuable metaphor time and time again. Giving birth has taught me how to cope with many of life's challenges.

Keeping an Open Mind

*Colleen was 31 years old and her husband, John,
was 38 when they had their first child at a hospital in
Princeton, New Jersey. They both work in managerial positions,
Colleen at a university, John in a state government
office. When Colleen went into labor three weeks
early, their baby was in the frank breech position.
She chose to deliver the baby vaginally.*

The obstetrics group in my town is composed of both obstetricians and midwives. They have been working together for about ten years, and many of the original doctors and midwives are still there. When you sign up with the group, you are given a choice of caretaker: obstetrician or midwife. I chose a midwife. I liked the noninterventionist philosophy of the midwives. I thought working with a midwife would give me the best chance of having the kind of birth experience that I had pictured. I was also interested in trying alternative methods for pain management.

214

My first child was due on February 1, 1994. As the Christmas holidays dragged by, I was growing bigger and more uncomfortable each day and was hoping that my baby would come early. I was excited when my appointment with the midwife early in January showed that I was 1 centimeter dilated. I was also pretty sure that I had already lost my mucous plug. I had passed something that actually looked like a big plug. However, since this was my first pregnancy, I wasn't sure.

My midwife confirmed with an ultrasound that my baby was still in the frank breech position (where the butt is presenting first and the legs are folded upward). She suggested that we arrange an "external version," in which the doctor tries to manually turn the baby through pressure applied to the abdomen. I was to meet the doctor at the hospital on Monday, January 10 for the external version.

January 9 was the day of my baby shower. I had just finished breakfast and was resting on the couch when I felt an unusual popping sensation in my lower abdomen. I felt just a little, tiny bit of leakage but since I'd been having "that" problem every time I sneezed, I just figured it was pregnancy incontinence. However, when I went to the bathroom I noticed a little trickle and started wondering if perhaps my water had broken.

I tried to remain calm and assured my husband, John, that I was positive it was nothing, but I called the midwife just to be sure. I still could not believe that my labor could be starting, even though in hindsight I realize that I had been feeling something similar to menstrual cramps for the past two days. I only knew at the time that I wasn't feeling anything at all like what I imagined contractions would feel like. My midwife,

Bobbie, asked me to come to the hospital so she could check me, and I told her I'd be there in about an hour. I still wanted to get ready for the baby shower at my mother's house. I was very much in denial.

While I was showering, I noticed that the cramps were getting more uncomfortable. When a baby is in frank breech position, cervical dilation is slow because the presenting part of the baby is too soft to stimulate effective contractions. However, once the water breaks, the buttocks are able to engage more, and then dilation begins in earnest. But even though I knew this, I refused to believe what was happening. I still laugh about the fact that when my husband and I left for the hospital, I told him not to bother bringing my bags because I was sure we'd be coming right home.

When we arrived at the hospital, Bobbie checked me and told me that yes, indeed, my water had broken, and this baby was coming. I wasn't quite 2 centimeters dilated yet, but since my water had broken, I was eligible to check in to the hospital. So I sent John home for the bags. Then I called my mother and told her I wouldn't be making it to the baby shower. She thought I was joking. It took some time to convince her that I actually was at the hospital and in labor.

Bobbie did an ultrasound, which confirmed that the baby was still in the breech position. In retrospect, I see that I wasn't very concerned about correct procedure, or even how I would be able to vaginally deliver a baby in frank breech position. But I didn't have much time to worry, since my water had broken so soon. Also, a month earlier, my sister had experienced exactly the same scenario, and had delivered her child vaginally without any problems.

According to the guidelines of our medical group, the frank breech position meant that I was required to have both a midwife and a doctor present for the birth. The doctor came in to consult with us. He explained that because of the baby's breech presentation, I could schedule a C-section and have the baby right away. I told him that I didn't want a cesarean but that my worst fear was to go through 15 hours of painful labor only to end up having a cesarean anyway.

The doctor questioned my resolve to go through with a vaginal delivery and pushed for the cesarean. At this point, Bobbie asked to speak with the doctor outside of the examination room. She had been in the group practice for a long time. She was well liked and respected, and she knew how and when to challenge the doctors.

When they came back into the room, Bobbie suggested that I wait and see how my labor progressed before making a decision about major surgery. The doctor agreed with her recommendation, and we all decided to give it some time.

It was now about 10:30 a.m. While I waited in bed in the examining room for John to get back with my bags, I started feeling very nauseated. The cramps were now beginning to feel more like contractions. The pains were very sharp and low in my abdomen: it felt like my abdomen was in a vice. I thought I was in a lot of pain then, but it was nothing compared to what was coming. When John returned, at Bobbie's insistence we walked the hospital corridors for over an hour while they prepared a room for us. When a contraction hit, I would stop and rock back and forth, which helped to get me through the worst of it. The nausea subsided after the first couple of hours.

Finally the nurses moved me into the private Labor and Delivery suite. It was a very comfortable room, with attractive wall hangings and furniture. We turned on the TV and I was happy when I realized I wouldn't have to miss the NFL playoff games that day after all. Bobbie came in to examine me and saw I was progressing, but slowly. I was dilated to 3 or 4 centimeters.

I tried to walk some more but soon was in too much pain to leave the room and just walked from one end of it to the other. The nurses would periodically put me on the monitor to check the baby and my contractions. Then they started an IV drip that I pulled along with me. Soon Bobbie suggested using Pitocin to help move things along. She didn't want me to labor so long that I was exhausted. She also knew that I was apprehensive about laboring for hours and ending up with a C-section. So, the Pitocin seemed like a fine idea. I was agreeable to anything that would help to speed up labor: I didn't care if it brought on stronger contractions.

By 2:00 p.m., I was unable to walk anymore, so Bobbie pulled in a rocking chair from the nurse's station and I rocked through the contractions. John stood behind me, rubbing my shoulders and massaging my head and temples with very hard pressure during the worst of the contractions. This helped tremendously. After each contraction I could relax. I stayed rocking in the chair all afternoon, only lying on the bed when Bobbie came in to examine me and monitor my progress. Lying on my back was excruciating. I didn't ask for medication and to this day I have no idea why. Maybe I was sure that nothing would stop this pain except Ryan being born.

At about 7:00 p.m. I was at 7 centimeters. Bobbie kept increasing the Pitocin, and finally, when she checked me at 9:00 p.m., she said I was at 9 centimeters. At 9:30, I felt a sudden change in my body during the contractions. It was a very strong pressure and an urge to push. I felt as though my body would push the baby out on its own, without my cooperation. The feeling was overwhelming, and I asked Bobbie to check me because I thought it was time to push. "Yes!" she said, "Push!"

RYAN SLID OUT SO EASILY THAT BOBBIE ALMOST DROPPED HIM.

It felt good to push—well, it hurt less anyway. The doctor came in to check on me. Bobbie had me demonstrate a push for him. I think she wanted him to see that I could do it. I pushed for about 20 minutes in the Labor and Delivery room, and then they took me to the operating room as a precaution since it was a breech birth.

In the operating room, I had a whole group of people observing. I suppose it was because of the breech birth, but I was too busy to take it all in. Looking back, I find it strange that this didn't bother me. I'm normally a very modest person. The doctor wanted Bobbie to catheterize me, but she told him she didn't think it was necessary. He did make her perform a very large episiotomy. After she gave me a shot of local anesthetic, I remember she cut some, then looked at him, and he indicated she should cut more. I felt nothing and was glad to make it as easy as possible for the baby to come out. I pushed for about 20 more minutes, and Ryan was born at 10:19 p.m., butt first. He slid out so easily that

219

Bobbie almost dropped him. She put him on my stomach and it was then I realized our baby was a boy.

John and I were ecstatic. The feeling of joy is as indescribable as the feeling of relief that the contractions are finally over. In fact, my first question to Bobbie after Ryan emerged was, "The contractions are over, right? That's it? No more?" The placenta came very quickly: I don't even remember pushing it out.

FIND A DOCTOR OR MIDWIFE YOU TRUST COMPLETELY, AND THEN TRUST HIM OR HER TO DO THE JOB.

Bobbie stitched the episiotomy, and then they wheeled my son and me back to our room. Ryan was 7 pounds, 11 ounces, with a great set of lungs. He really looked funny. We affectionately called him "Butt-Head" because his legs were splayed out with his feet up by his ears from being in the frank breech position for so long. For the next week or so, we had to continually pull and stretch his legs to strengthen his muscles and reposition his legs.

I didn't sleep at all that night, and even though he went home, I don't think John got much sleep either. We were just too excited. Ryan, however, slept soundly until the next morning. He was a very sleepy baby, the kind you have to wake up to feed.

The most important thing I have learned after having two children is that you cannot have a preconceived notion of your birth experience. My advice is to try to keep an open mind and remember that each birth experience is unique. It's okay to have your preferences, but don't rule anything out. Find a doctor or midwife you trust completely, and then trust him or her to do the job.

After delivering my second child vaginally in the normal birth position, I can tell you I prefer breech. It is much more difficult and painful to have that giant head pushing down there for so long. I will always remember how tiny and smooth Ryan's behind was coming out, compared to my second child's big head.

P.S. I remember nothing at all about the football games.

The Very Fine Edge
of My Limits

When Megan and Mark's first child was born,
Megan was 32 years old and Mark was 33.
After three and a half years of infertility treatments and two
miscarriages, they conceived this baby and carried it to term.
They are both astrophysicists, and at the time of the baby's birth,
they were both looking for jobs. Their baby was born in a hospital
in Baltimore, Maryland, the city where they now work.

On February 4, at around 7:30 p.m., I was chasing my dog around the living room when my water suddenly broke. Even though I was nine months pregnant, I was surprised. I immediately phoned my midwife and the future grandparents. Since my water had broken, my midwife told me, as a precaution against infection, not to get into a tub (which I really, really wanted to do) but to instead try showering once the contractions began.

Within an hour, I had gone directly into "active labor," with contractions about 50 to 70 seconds in length and two and a half to three minutes apart. Once they began, my husband flew around getting the suitcase, setting up the car, and checking in with the midwife, while I got into the shower.

Unfortunately, a shower was inadequate for the job: it was a cold, cold day, only 10 degrees outside, with 30-mile-per-hour winds, and our house was chilly. The shower only warmed a little patch of skin, so I had to get out. At this point, the contractions felt like super-intense menstrual cramps, but they were getting stronger with each one. This scared me.

Fluid kept gushing out of me. I tried using diapers so I could walk around without messing up the rug, but I felt really uncomfortable. I hung out on the toilet, so the water would drip in there, but that was not a fun place to be either. My butt actually got numb after a while.

Next, I started to vomit. Sometimes my vomiting overlapped a contraction. This was distressing because I felt like I couldn't concentrate on anything.

Sometime after 10:00 p.m., my husband called the midwife with the details of what was going on, and after some conversation, we all agreed it was time to meet at the hospital.

The 30-minute drive to the hospital was awful. Poor Mark. He listened patiently to me complain during the entire drive. Now the contractions were consistently about 90 seconds long, with a strong sudden peak, and then a gradual decrease in intensity. My daydreams about what to expect in my first labor had never included kneeling in a parking lot at 11:00 at night, being pierced by icy winds in 10-degree temperatures. I have to admit, though, I wasn't feeling the cold much at all. Instead I was wishing I could be on another planet.

Once in the hospital, another contraction stopped me on my way to the birthing room. I had to pause and kneel on the hallway floor. Mark and a security guard pushing an empty wheelchair were following me. I had declined to use the chair because at the time sitting did not seem like a good idea. Lying in a hot tub seemed like a good idea.

The mandatory fetal scan showed that all was well, and an examination revealed that although I was dilated only 3 centimeters, the baby was well positioned.

Dilation did not proceed quickly, despite my hope that multi-peaked, long, intense contractions early in the process meant a speedy labor. I was put on an IV immediately to prevent dehydration because I was still vomiting between contractions. Throughout my labor, I had ice chips but I couldn't keep anything else down. The birthing room contained a Jacuzzi, which I used and which helped me in between contractions, but the contractions themselves I felt full force. Going to the bathroom was tough, because every time I released the flow of urine, I'd be smacked by another contraction—wham!—right there.

Drugs were starting to seem like a really good idea. But I took this as a good sign that I might be near the end, so instead I asked for more ice chips and along I went. I experimented with moaning; this both helped and didn't help. It seemed to take away from my concentration rather than relax my body. I may have also felt a little cultural inhibition. I am the strong, silent type, so groaning seems like complaining to me.

When I wanted the Jacuzzi to be hotter but that wasn't allowed, it became less appealing. Finally, I got out of the tub and spent the next three or four hours sitting in a semireclined chair, sort of in a trance state. I imagined running endless track intervals; I imagined horses giving birth; I imagined barren, swirling desert planets with red dust; I imagined the universe in all its emptiness sucking me out toward the stars. All this seemed to help. But the contractions, which felt like I was being sucked in and out of a rolling press, crunching my bones, were getting even more intense. I felt like I was being pushed to the very fine edge of my limits.

My husband was the person I looked to after each contraction for comfort and stability. My midwife dozed a little during the latter part of the first stage of labor, but Mark stayed awake and focused on my face the whole time. That was important to me. Every time a contraction stopped, I would look at his face. I felt like I needed a validation of the process, someone to confirm that this was real, that I was still alive, and that what I was going through

EVERY TIME A CONTRACTION STOPPED, I WOULD LOOK AT MY HUSBAND'S FACE. I FELT LIKE I NEEDED A VALIDATION OF THE PROCESS, SOMEONE TO CONFIRM THAT THIS WAS REAL, THAT I WAS STILL ALIVE, AND THAT WHAT I WAS GOING THROUGH WAS IMPORTANT.

was important. He was my anchor. He isn't a touchy-feely kind of person, so he had to be coached a little bit to press on my lower back to help with the pain, but he worked very hard at it, and that really helped.

Again, the drug option seemed like a really, really good idea. I panicked at the thought that I might no longer have this option, that I had waited too long. With my approval, the midwife gave me a shot of something, and I moved to the birthing bed. The shot did not affect the pain at all, but at least I was not panicked anymore. I was now about 7 centimeters dilated.

Once I was on the bed, I started moaning involuntarily. Mark coached me to keep the moans low-pitched and not to say "No," but instead to say more positive words like "Out" (which, of course, disintegrated into "Owww!"). Eventually, I started grunting involuntarily at the peak of each contraction. The midwife quickly checked me and told me not to push yet, that I still had a lip of cervix in the way; but I overheard her telling my husband not to restrict me from pushing at the peak of the contractions, as that might help to complete my dilation.

Then, I saw progress. The pediatric nurse started setting up her tools. "A good sign," I thought. The dawn started to pink the skies over Baltimore—we had a panoramic view from the 16th floor of the hospital. The bed was very high, so I could see straight out the window. I felt like I was at the end of a long night's work (my profession often entails all-night observations), and that helped me a lot. Then, the lip of the cervix went away, and they said I could push. Mark got behind me and held me more upright.

Pushing was the best part. It took me an hour and a half, but I hardly felt the contractions because now I could push during them. Then the contractions got further apart, and I started to anticipate them so I could hurry this baby on out. I pushed around the head for what seemed like a long time, and the midwife said, "I know you didn't want an episiotomy, but there's a lot of skin here and I think it would help." She had a mirror set up by this point, so I took a look and I saw exactly what she meant, so I agreed. Later, the midwife said that what I had couldn't really be called an episiotomy, it was so small, only 1 centimeter or so, and only skin. I hardly noticed it during recovery. It itched a little as it healed, but compared to what I was trying to avoid (a muscle cut), it was nothing.

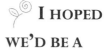 **I HOPED WE'D BE A NATURAL BREASTFEEDING TEAM. BUT I HAD TROUBLE.**

With the very next push, the baby flew out. I swear her head and body just flew out. I was saying to myself, "Ow, Ow, Ow!" but I was so excited and tired, it was really great. It was all over and now here was this slimy baby! Mark leaned over, asking what it was, and the midwife said, "See for yourself." He said, "It's a girl!" and I was one happy mama! Mark was completely overwhelmed and crying. He got to cut the cord. Delivery of the placenta came with another one or two pushes.

I wanted to nurse Michaela right away, and I tried to get her latched on myself. I hoped we'd be a natural breastfeeding team. But I had trouble. My midwife stepped in and pinched my nipple, hard. I gasped in surprise at how hard she had yanked on my nipple, but I was relieved to see some colostrum come out. Michaela latched on and I had my first lesson in breastfeeding. I wasn't used to that kind of pressure on my nipples, and for me, it was not very pleasant. Michaela nursed for 10 minutes while I gritted my teeth. In fact, for the first few

227

weeks, breastfeeding was a toe-curling experience for me but eventually, with advice from everyone I knew, and a lot of patience and perseverance, it worked out very well for both of us.

Michaela Rachel was born February 5, 1995, the coldest day of the year in Baltimore, at 9:27 a.m., weighing 6 pounds, 14¾ ounces. I had been in labor for 13½ hours, including at least 90 minutes of pushing. Since it was important to us that at least one of us be with her at all times, Mark followed Michaela around during the preliminary check-up procedure and the brief visit to the nursery for an examination by the pediatrician. After that, Michaela was with us for our entire hospital stay, including her subsequent pediatric examinations.

Now We Are a Family Again

Trisha was a 26-year-old social worker and her husband, Al,
was a 30-year-old database programmer in 1996
when they had their second baby via a second cesarean section.
They lived in Oakland, California. This birth was very special
for them because they had lost their first child
when she was three months old due to highly unusual
congenital heart problems.

At my 32-week appointment, we began to realize how large our baby was. The ultrasound suggested she was the size of an average 38-week fetus. Two years later (after the measurement standards had changed), I found out that I had actually had gestational diabetes, hence my baby's size. But at the time, since I was a large woman, fairly young, and testing within then-established parameters, we didn't look for a medical cause for her growth rate.

That 32-week appointment was the first time my obstetrician suggested we consider a C-section as the safest method for delivery of a baby that size, especially since we would want to wait a few more weeks to insure that her lungs were fully developed, and by then she would be even larger.

I was very disappointed, as I had very much looked forward to a VBAC (vaginal birth after cesarean). I hung on to some hope, but week after week the baby continued to grow. When she was an estimated 10 pounds at week 38, we had to face the inevitable. After lots of thought and research, we decided to take my doctor's advice and we scheduled the C-section for Monday, October 23, during my 39th week. At her size, the risks of a vaginal delivery were just not something we would have been comfortable with, and it would likely have been a long and scary labor. I know that lots of large babies are delivered vaginally, but I wasn't up to the anguish if she got stuck. After losing our first child, Al and I needed this birth to go especially smoothly. For our emotional peace of mind, I had had an amniocentesis done at 18 weeks, and also an in utero electrocardiogram, so we knew we had a healthy baby girl this time, and we decided our priority was to deliver her safely.

We had to be at the hospital at 5:30 a.m. for the presurgery preparations. I'm not a morning person and told Al that it was only because I wanted this baby so much that I would consider getting up at 4:30. I had lots of heartburn the night before, but wasn't allowed to eat or drink anything—not even water—due to the fasting requirements before the surgery. I was very tired, but I wasn't very sleepy. I was running on pure excitement. As we drove to the hospital, we both were in shock, unable to believe that soon we would have a healthy baby.

There was only one laboring woman in the maternity ward that morning, so we received lots of attention getting prepped. Al and I were so happy and joyous, and apparently a little loud, that we attracted a stream of visitors. Nurses and staff kept dropping by our room to chat.

The first thing the nurse did in preparation was to try to print a monitoring strip of the baby's heartbeat. Well, the baby was kicking so much that the monitoring belt on my abdomen could not detect a regular heartbeat, and the nurse had to move it around quite a bit to get the printout she needed. At least we had no question about the baby's vigor.

Next, my belly and upper pubic hair were shaved in preparation for the bikini-cut, and then I was given an IV. The IV bottle was hung on a portable frame so I could wheel it around with me.

During this time, I began to lose my confidence and become anxious. Perhaps it was because it was all happening so slowly. My first C-section had been an emergency and had frightened me quite a bit, and then, three months later, I had lost the baby. Now, going through the procedure in a kind of slow motion gave me time to consider what was happening and brought back my fears from the first time. I wondered if I really would be so lucky as to have a healthy child.

The anesthesiologist came to talk to me before the surgery, which was scheduled for 7:30 a.m. He was just wonderful. He reassured me that it's normal to feel as if you can't breathe during the procedure, something that had frightened me the last time. He explained that the numbing goes so far up your chest that it affects the muscles surrounding your diaphragm and you feel as if it isn't expanding. He told me he

231

would count my breaths for me aloud if I needed reassurance during the procedure. His warm manner and thorough approach helped to calm me down.

It also helped that we had written a birth plan for the staff, telling them about our first child and what we hoped for this baby during our stay. All the Labor and Delivery and most of the postpartum nurses read it, and many cried. They understood why we did not want to be separated from our child for even a moment, if possible. We even wanted to give her her first bath together.

A student nurse was on rotation that morning and this was his first birth. He wound up staying with us from the prep through the surgery. He cried when our baby was born and told us he was grateful that this was his introduction to childbirth.

Just before the surgery, my doctor came in to chat with us and expressed her concern about how I was doing emotionally. She joked with us, which relieved some of the tension, and basically let me know that she knew it was hard for me.

At 7:30 a.m., wheeling my IV beside me, I walked into the operating room, something I had not expected to do. That made me feel strong. I took a few moments to look closely at my surroundings. The room was tiny and so was the operating table. It was very narrow and its height could be adjusted to accommodate the height of the primary physician. My OB is a short woman, so the table was rather low. I had a chance to study the dizzying array of gleaming equipment. Trays draped in blue cloths held various instruments. A suction unit, which they use to remove your amniotic fluids and blood after the baby is born, stood in one corner. There were monitors set up for the anesthesiologist to observe my vital signs and a respirator for the baby—a standard piece of equipment, just in case. And I saw a large white bulletin board with my name written on it in capital letters. That made me feel like I owned the room.

The room was crowded. Not only was it full of equipment, but it also held 13 people, counting me and Al: three scrub nurses; my OB and her partner; our doula, Debbie, by our special request; the student nurse; a Labor and Delivery nurse; our pediatrician (also by our special request); the nurse anesthetist (required by California state law to examine the baby after surgery); and the anesthesiologist.

When the anesthesiologist came in, he explained all the monitors to me. Meanwhile, the nurse velcroed an automatic blood pressure cuff to my one free arm (the other one had the IV in it). The cuff was distracting because periodically and without warning it inflates and takes your blood pressure. While the anesthesiologist inserted the spinal block, he talked me through each step of the process, which I appreciated, and my OB stood in front of me, reassuring me. I had to sit on the side of the table, legs dangling, and curl over for the doctor to insert the needle into the small of my back. He did this easily, and the effect of the spinal was immediate. Within one or two seconds, I collapsed and fell backward into the waiting arms of the nurses. A spinal block goes deeper into your spine than an epidural, so the drug is delivered immediately. Also the numbing is more extensive—from chest to pubic bone. I did not find the procedure frightening at all. I was just impressed that they managed to catch me as I fell.

After the drip was started, Al and Debbie, whom we'd engaged before we knew I'd be having a C-section, came in. They were in scrubs like the rest of the team, wearing blue caps and blue shoe covers. Debbie had brought her camera, and the doctor helped her figure out where to shoot from for the best pictures. Someone told the doctor I really wanted to see the baby be born, and the anesthesiologist produced a large hand mirror he keeps around for women like me. He would have held it for me, too, but Al decided he'd rather have him do anesthesiologist things, like watch my monitors. When the time came, Al held the mirror for me and did a darn good job, too.

BECAUSE I COULDN'T FEEL ANYTHING, IT WAS LIKE WATCHING SOMEONE ELSE GIVE BIRTH.

The anesthesiologist stood behind my head, with one of his monitors beside him, and Al stood to the right of my head, Debbie to the left. Everyone else came in rather quickly and stood on the other side of the drape they had set up to block my view.

At this point, I became pretty distracted by the extremely odd feeling of not being able to feel anything much past my breasts. I felt as if I were floating, having an out-of-body experience. Because I couldn't feel anything, it was like watching someone else give birth.

Within minutes of everyone assembling, Al told me, "Trish, they are cutting already." He was so excited. Before long, he practically shouted, "There's fluid—and it's clear!" Seeing healthy-looking fluid was a good sign. He told me later that when they cut the sac, fluid spurted up and out.

It took much longer than I expected to get the baby out. My doctor later apologized because she forgot to tell me that with repeat sections, there's scar tissue to go through, so it takes a lot longer, as some tissues have adhered to one another and the layers aren't quite so easy to cut through. Eventually, the scar tissue breaks down and dissolves, but mine was only a year old, so there was still quite a bit.

It only took them an extra three or four minutes, but to me, it felt like an eternity. I began to panic, certain that I would somehow stop breathing. In retrospect, I think that I panicked as I became aware of the reality: I was powerless in this situation where I couldn't feel anything. So I focused on the one thing I could still control: my breathing. The anesthesiologist noticed the wild look in my eyes, put his hands on my shoulders, and kept talking to me very calmly. This helped. Debbie and Al were holding my hands. I looked up at Al, standing by my side, and I couldn't help but feel his excitement and joy—it was pouring from him. That made me feel much better.

Once the incision was made, my OB reached into the sac up to her elbow, hooked her hand around the baby's butt, and tried to pull her out. At the same time, her partner began to push on my fundus (the top of the uterus) to assist. But the baby was so large, they had trouble getting her out. Al was holding the mirror for me and I was peering at it, trying to see what was going on. Rather thankfully, I could not see into the big hole in my lower abdomen, but mostly saw the bulge of my tummy and a hint of what was on the other side. I saw my tummy ripple as my OB's partner pushed down on me again and again. I was vaguely aware of the fact that they seemed to be having trouble. My

OB's partner actually had to get up and put one knee on the table in order to lean his shoulder into my fundus and push much harder. The anesthesiologist even reached across my chest and tried to push from behind the drape, though I don't think he had much effect. My doctor told me later (and this is where Al and I just crack up) that they almost couldn't get her out. She was stuck, even with a C-section! It seems that because of the previous scar tissue, they hadn't been able to cut a bigger-than-usual incision (which they had wanted to do since they expected her to be unusually large), so they had to kind of squish her out. It was very disconcerting for me to be squeezed so much and still not feel anything. And I was mad because the doctor was blocking my view.

Finally, the OB got down from the table, and all my attention was on the mirror, watching my belly squish down. All of a sudden, a wet head with a shocking thatch of dark hair appeared. It was so neat to see her come out. I was told later that my view looked just about how it looks when you have a vaginal birth. Al told me later that he heard a whimpering then, before she was fully born. I was thinking about how dark her hair was and how much there was of it—and how incredible this all was. Her face looked just like those faces in the birthing films from childbirth classes. She was pink and wet and sleek. I don't know quite how to describe it, but all of a sudden, I knew it was okay and that my dream had come true. I noticed that she had an awfully big head, especially in comparison to my petite, 5-foot-1-inch doctor's hands as she held it. The doctors paused here to suction her—to clear her mouth and throat. Within seconds, I saw the rest of the body pop out. She flashed by in the mirror as the doctor pulled her all the way out and they started to dry her off.

She cried right away. My impression at the time was that she cried before her feet even cleared the incision. I was amazed by the strength of her voice.

My doctor stepped right back after they had cut the bulk of the cord from me and walked around the drape with the baby, just as she had promised me she would do. To me, she was beautiful even with lots of her umbilical cord still attached. I had told my doctor ahead of time that I needed to see her with lots of her cord, so that I would feel like this was the same baby I had grown. The cord was so thick and strong looking (and long!) when it went by in the mirror. And there it was, hanging from her. I *had* made this baby. Wow! I reached out, unable to hold back, and grasped Gwen's foot. The doctor became alarmed and told me I couldn't touch her just yet because, with my abdominal cavity open, they had to be very cautious about contamination, and my hand was not sterile. (Ironically, I was the only one in the room who wasn't scrubbed and sterile.) But you could see that under her mask the doctor was grinning from ear to ear. She and Al drifted over to do the hand-off to our pediatrician, who was waiting in the corner of the room.

Gwen was still crying and the sound continued to fill the room. She sounded so mad. I was amazed that she could cry so loudly for so long.

While they delivered the placenta and started the long task of cleaning me and putting me back together, I was craning my neck toward the warming table where my baby was. (Did you know they actually take your uterus out to clean it? They lay it on your belly or some such. I didn't watch. I can't quite decide if I wish I had seen that part . . .) I looked away from my baby long enough to see the placenta.

They brought it over to me in a bowl. Boy, was it enormous, and very red!

Next, I heard the pediatrician say, "Eight and nine." My labor coach made sure I had heard those Apgar numbers. I was pleased, but the baby was still crying loudly. Soon, she quieted down and I found out why. Al walked over to me, holding her in a blanket. He looked at me and said something. I couldn't tell what he was trying to say, his voice was so choked up. I had to have him repeat it twice.

What he had been saying, it turned out, was, "Does she look like a Gwen, then?" He wanted to name her right away, to use her name. He was trembling and crying, he was so excited. I thanked the universe that had let my husband be so happy finally. He had been devastated by the loss of our first child. He held our new baby so I could see her and I just marveled at her little face. Debbie took a picture that has to be from that very moment.

Then Al and Gwen left for the recovery room across the hall. The operating rooms are kept rather cold so bacteria will have less of a chance to grow, and we were all so entranced, the medical staff included, that we had kept her there a bit too long, and she was getting chilled. It was time to get her out of there and get back to business.

At that point, I wanted to just withdraw into my body. I was frustrated because I couldn't hold my daughter, or touch her, or examine her. And I was awfully sick of not being able to feel my body. A C-section takes about 45 minutes to perform. The birth, from spinal to delivery, is less than 15 minutes of that time. The rest is cleaning and stitching the uterus, and stapling the abdomen. So I was also bored. Now that I knew Gwen was okay, I just wanted it to be over. I closed my eyes and felt as if I could go to sleep, which made my doula a bit nervous. But the anesthesiologist was not concerned: the spinal has this effect on most people. Finally they were done.

Somewhere in the middle of this, someone poked his head back in and told us all what she weighed: 11 pounds, 1 ounce! There were gasps and laughs. It turns out everyone had been taking bets from the moment we all saw her as to how big Gwen actually was. Al says that when they put her on the scale and it registered over 11 pounds, he found it hard to believe, but he knew I would be happy. I was surprised, but the news made me feel even better. I had been saying that if I had to go through another C-section because they thought the baby was big, she had better *be* big! Now I felt at peace with having missed a vaginal birth and having had to relive the fear and anxiety of the first C-section.

As they were preparing to transfer me from the operating table to the gurney, the anesthesiologist stepped back from the table for a moment. All of a sudden I felt something odd happening, like an awkward lurch, and I felt my body shifting to the left side. Debbie looked startled, and I asked what had happened. The anesthesiologist laughed and said, "Sheesh, I step away for a moment . . ." Turns out, my leg had fallen off the table and I had started to slide toward the edge of it—yikes! Then several people rolled and pushed me onto the gurney. It was an odd sensation as I was still incapable of feeling anything—it was hard to feel that I was moving, let alone being touched. Finally, I was wheeled out and across the hall to the recovery room and made comfortable.

Al was there with Gwen, chuckling to her in a distinctive way that he still does. Someone cranked up the head of the gurney a bit (breaking the rules, as you are supposed to remain flat in the recovery room following a C-section), and I then could see her, all sweet and pink. Soon I was holding her, and I felt like I had entered a special place in Heaven. She was smacking her lips, and I responded by putting a finger in her mouth. She sucked and hard, too. One of the nurses observed this, and all of a sudden, she was helping me get Gwen in the right position, and before I knew it, Gwen was nursing. I didn't know how the world could get better. I realized at that moment that to nurse a baby is what I had really wanted, and Gwen had just opened up her little mouth, I had somehow gotten my nipple in there, and wow, we were doing it! I think I may have cried. The odd thing was that I could feel the pressure of her body on my lower chest, but I could not feel her skin on my skin—I was still totally under the anesthesia when I nursed her.

We hung out in the recovery room for what seemed like forever. After an hour or two, I wanted to get to a phone and tell the world about how Al and I had entered some weird twilight zone where everything was perfect.

After my vital signs had been stable for the required amount of time, I was transferred to my room. For a small additional charge, we could have a private room, so we decided it was worth the money. The time in the hospital was mostly just fine. Al (who stayed the whole time) and I sat around in awe. It was glorious to see Al being Super Dad, able to calm Gwen with a single snuggle. He got a little panicked that first night when she was upset because she was hungry, but all in all he made the experience everything I dreamed of. Had it not been for him, I would have had to put her in the well-baby nursery at night so I could get some rest, and if I had had to be separated from my newborn, I would have been one incredibly bummed-out woman. As it was, we were only apart once, for those few minutes while they stitched me up.

I recovered from the surgery quickly. I never needed the strongest painkillers they offered, though I did struggle a bit with pain, especially the second day, after all the anesthesia wore off.

We came home two days after Gwen was born. All together. The three of us. Al and I had a hard time believing it. When our pediatrician came into our hospital room that morning and pronounced Gwen quite healthy and able to go home, Al and I did the only logical thing. We stared at each other, stared at her, and both burst into tears. We were still not adjusted to the reality of our success.

But now we are. Gwen is a sloppy eater, and when she comes off my breast, there is milk all around her face and dripping out of her mouth. I happily wipe it away, glad there is so much that I can waste a few drops. She doesn't like to open her mouth wide, so it makes getting her latched on right a somewhat tricky thing, but really, it's been so easy. And such a joy! Just as I had thought, she makes the C-section a dust mote in the past.

MICHAEL'S BIRTH

A Close Call (1966)

Idrian and Jane were living in Dar es Salaam, Tanzania
at the time of their son's birth in 1966. Jane was working as an
economist and Idrian was a professor of economics.
Idrian writes, "I think it is important to remember that in 1966,
men were not very in touch with their emotions. We certainly
did not have sophisticated names for all the variations.
So, while I have tried to accurately revisit those feelings,
I have kept them relatively simple; as they were at the time."

"I think my water's broken," my wife, Jane, said.

"Shhhhh!" came several indignant voices from the darkened theater at the University of Dar es Salaam in Tanzania. I can't remember what we were watching that last day of August 1966. I do remember the shot of fear that hit first my heart, then my chest. Here? Right here? In the movies? What was I to do? I was worried that my "shhsh-ing" faculty colleagues were surely going to next hiss: "Go outside and have your baby!"

Back in our home, I had to keep moving while the university's Swedish doctor examined Jane in the bedroom. Economics professors were supposed to be smart, but I felt dumb. It was six weeks before Jane's due date, we had done everything we were supposed to do, and now this was happening. Maybe Jane's job as an economist for the Tanzanian Government had been too much for her. Or maybe my trip home months earlier to finish my Ph.D. dissertation had been a mistake. "What do I do now?" I thought. "How can I make this come out all right?" I was frustrated and worried but my mind was blank.

It was a relatively cool night for Africa but I was lathered, caught between the sounds of the gigantic bullfrogs, who seemed to be barking their disapproval from dark places, and wondering whether this doctor, who had spent 20 years in the bush treating malaria and gastrointestinal diseases, knew what he was doing. In Africa, midwives delivered babies.

"Your wife is not very dilated," said the doctor, "but her water has broken. When the pains are less than five minutes apart, drive her to hospital." He had his sleeves rolled up but I saw no rubber gloves. Nor had he called for boiling water or clean towels, so how could he know how dilated she was?

More than a full day later, around midnight, as we were playing Scrabble and recording contractions, Jane cried, "Ohhh! That was a good one. How long was it?"

I looked at my watch and wrote down the time in a column on our score sheet. "Jane: 176; Idrian: 133; Baby: 12:10 = 6 mins. 22 secs." After 30 hours of irregular labor pains, Jane was now exhausted, not so much from the pain as from the waiting and wondering if her fate was to remain in labor for the rest of her natural life.

243

"Maybe if I talk to her, she'll hurry up and come," I said. I was sure it was a girl.

I wanted to do something but felt helpless in the face of this momentous event. I bent forward. Jane was against the headboard of the bed, barely able to reach the Scrabble tiles over the watermelonlike bulge that had swollen her from below her breasts to the tops of her legs.

"Hurry up, little darlin'," I said against Jane's belly button. "Mommy's getting tired and Daddy can't wait to hold you!"

"Ugggg!" Jane grunted. "It worked! That was less than five minutes!"

It was my cue to take charge. Finally, there was something for me to do.

Getting to the hospital was no easy task. The passenger seat in our Volkswagen Beetle was as far back as it would go, but Jane's belly still seemed nearly against the glove compartment, and since she couldn't bend, there was no way she could fit into the tiny back seat. On the dark road with dim car lights, the eight miles of potholes was pure hell. Little did I suspect that it foreshadowed the nightmare ahead. I navigated around the pits like a slalom skier, the bright moon giving me just enough light to pick out the darker spots in the road. Still, the ride was a rugged one, and I almost thought I could hear the baby crying between Jane's brave grunts from labor pains and the thumps.

When we arrived at the Agha Kahn Hospital, it was dark. The empty parking lot and the tiny lobby were dark, too. As we waited for someone to answer our ring at the 10-foot wooden door into the hospital, I kept wondering whether we had done the right thing in deciding to have the baby in Africa. Up until now, it had seemed safe enough. After all, Africans had babies all the time. "But what if there is a problem?" I now wondered.

A Pakistani nurse whisked Jane into the faintly lighted hall of the maternity ward and promptly slammed the door in my face as if to say "Fathers not needed here!"

There were no chairs or benches, so I sat outside on the steps and listened to huge palm leaves clapping in the gentle ocean breeze. Over the months of Jane's pregnancy, I had moved from being the most important person in her life into second place. I was 30 years old and I could understand it. But I had been unsuccessful finding a new role for myself. I was unhappy sitting there. I wanted to help, but felt useless, replaced, and profoundly lonely.

Helper! That's it! I decided I would be the main helper. I wanted this baby more than I could say. If she was beautiful, I would protect her from marauding boys. If she was ugly, I would be her pal, hang out with her and take her places.

Nearly an hour later, the nurse came through the door and thrust a paper on a clipboard under my face.

"Sign, please!" she said. It was an order, not a request.

"What am I signing?"

"Permission to give oxygen to Mrs. R," she said offhandedly.

My alarm system flared. "Why do you need to give her oxygen?" I asked.

"Just sign. Don't ask questions. We are in charge here!"

"I won't sign anything unless you tell me what's going on," I insisted.

She sighed with an air that said: You will sign, regardless of my answer, so why are you wasting my time?

She said, "Baby's heart beating too quickly. We must give oxygen."

That did it. I was falling through a hole in the world. At the same moment I saw that I was now needed. I said, "I want to see the doctor. Now!"

"There is no doctor. A midwife is delivering Mrs. R's baby. I am the nurse in charge."

"Get a doctor!" I repeated. "There has to be one on duty in this hospital. I won't sign without talking to a doctor."

She disappeared, leaving me in the dark again. My mind began to race: What does this mean? Are we going to lose the baby? Is the umbilical cord wrapped around her neck? Was she somehow stuck in the birth canal? "Oh please let them be okay!" I prayed.

As I waited, I walked nervously back and forth. A full moon in the eastern sky lit up the tropical night and threw its beams off the calm waters of the Indian Ocean, about a hundred yards from where I paced. My shadow was cast along the floor and up the back wall. I couldn't stay still. I felt scared; I wanted to cry. An Indian doctor finally came and led me to an office.

"The baby is having a difficult time being born," she said. "It is in distress. The oxygen will go to the baby through Mrs. R and that will slow down its heart."

I signed the papers immediately. "Look, doctor, I want the truth," I said. "What's the worst thing that can happen?"

"The baby could be born dead," she said. In her voice, there was both trust and resignation. She knew I could handle the truth and that I knew how many babies had died in this, one of the 25 poorest countries in the world.

"I don't want to come back here and console my wife over a dead baby. I want to be with her," I said. "She needs me," I wanted to add. "And I need her!" How could they break us up now? We had been a team, had decided everything together, helped each other. Now I was on the outside, feeling helpless.

"All right," the doctor agreed, "but you are not to tell her why we are giving oxygen."

In the labor room, Jane lay on a hospital gurney. There were no stirrups and the surface did not look wide enough for her body. The walls were marked and badly in need of paint. The light was pale and the floor and sink looked anything but antiseptic. An African midwife had her hands on Jane's abdomen, as if she were trying to push the baby out. A thin oxygen tube was threaded into Jane's nose.

The midwife looked disapprovingly at me, but accepted the doctor's instructions in Swahili that I be allowed to stay. Jane smiled bravely. Hot tears streamed down my cheeks as I took her hand. I wanted the baby a lot, but I wanted Jane to be okay even more. I felt all my bravery rolling out of my eyes.

"It's okay," she soothed. "Everything's going to be fine."

I felt ashamed that she was comforting me. I tried to reach deeper inside myself, for something I could give her. The midwife, who had not taken her eyes off me in the few minutes I had been there, said, "You go. No good you here. No good for memsahib."

She was right. I was taking more than I was giving. I left and dragged my deeply depressed soul along the dark corridor, through the great door, and out again, into the moonlit night. I drove along the pot-holed roads to a friend's apartment.

AT 4:30 A.M., I HEARD A TINY CRY AND KNEW THAT, AFTER 36 HOURS OF LABOR, JANE HAD DELIVERED A LIVE BABY. NO SOUND, BEFORE OR SINCE, HAS SO GLADDENED ME.

That was the worst time of my life. Instead of pacing and worrying, like typical expectant fathers, here I was expecting my baby to die. We had already aborted one pregnancy when Jane had contracted German measles in the first month. That had brought about months of depression for both of us. How was it possible to lose another baby? And so far from home. We had lots of friends in Tanzania but they could not make up for our families, thousands of miles away.

They had told me to come back to the hospital in five hours. That would be at 6:00 a.m. This time I could not manage to avoid the holes in the road, but I was driving so slowly that it didn't matter much. Everything felt like lead inside me, and I could not stop my mind from composing death telegrams for our relatives back home. The pain was so great that at times I felt separated from my body, as if I were watching myself, wondering how I could survive such a loss, and how I would be able to carry Jane through it. I felt alone, discarded, abandoned by

Jane, needy of the attention she was getting, wanting someone to talk to, bitterly cognizant of my uselessness because I was a man. I had fathered this child and shared Jane's pregnancy, yet in this hour of despair, I had nowhere to go with my needs. In fact, I felt deeply ashamed that I even had them.

After two hours with no sleep, I drove back to the hospital to wait in the nurse's office. At 4:30 a.m., I heard a tiny cry and knew that, after 36 hours of labor, Jane had delivered a live baby. No sound, before or since, has so gladdened me. On the edge of darkness, I was suddenly whooshed into a galaxy of joy.

Now I would be able to begin forging the place in his life that I could not find in his birth. Six days later our son, Michael, and Jane came home.

Running Up Mount Everest

Paula, an editor, was 28 years old, and her husband,
Ian, an acupuncturist, was 26, when they had their first child,
as planned, at home. They had been married a little over two
years at the time and were living in Seattle, where Ian
was studying naturopathic medicine.

My pregnancy had been a joy. I was extremely tired the first three months, but from the fourth month on, I was full of energy. I was a woman who washed the walls. I also enjoyed the fact that I could eat to my heart's content, and though I gained 45 pounds, it was all in my belly.

My husband and I had agreed that we wanted our child to be born at home. It seemed the most logical place to us. When I was pregnant, I made a point of becoming as familiar as possible with the entire birth process. I spoke to others who had home births and became convinced that given my healthy pregnancy, there was no reason not to have the baby in the comfort of my own home, with my friends around me. My father was not comfortable with my choice at all, but my mom, who is from Holland, where home birth is a matter of course, was supportive and expressed envy at the options available to me.

We began to look for a caregiver, and everyone we spoke with asked us if we had interviewed Molly, so we decided to meet her. Molly is a naturopathic physician as well as a licensed midwife, with many years of home-birth experience, so we knew her credentials were good. But I was convinced she was the right caregiver for me the moment I spoke to her. Something just clicked and I liked her immediately.

I was due on my husband's birthday, which was also the night of his last clinic shift—he was completing his training as a naturopathic physician. Since this was my first child, I expected to go past my due date, and I stayed up late to celebrate with Ian. We didn't go to bed until midnight.

After maybe two hours of sleep that night, I started having pains I couldn't sleep through, approximately every seven minutes. They were very much like menstrual cramps, only my abdomen also became painfully rigid. I guessed that my labor had arrived.

At around 7:00 a.m., when the pains started coming exactly five minutes apart and stayed that way for an hour, I stopped giving the play-by-play to Ian and paged Molly, who sent over her student, Elizabeth, to check my progress. I couldn't believe after the intensity of the contractions I was only 2 centimeters dilated and 90 percent effaced.

By 10:00 a.m., the contractions were coming every two minutes like clockwork. But I didn't feel ready to give birth yet. I felt I had so much to do, like clean the apartment and shop—I didn't feel like doing anything sensible, like sleeping. I was too excited for that.

251

At about 11:00, I insisted Ian take me to the grocery store, where I proceeded to give the staff heart failure by having contractions up against the walls, on the shopping cart, at the checkout counter. Then I went home and started vacuuming, something I desperately wanted to do for some reason, even though Molly had told me to get into bed in order to conserve my strength for the long haul ahead.

By now, my friend Christine had arrived. She made me eat some pasta, which I could only do in between contractions. I remember laughing a great deal.

I spent the next few hours, until about 4:00 p.m., either in the bathtub soaking or out of it calling my friends back home in Montreal. At this point, I had precisely one minute to talk at a time, as my contractions were regular and very intense. Each telephone conversation was basically, "Hi, I'm in labor, uh-oh, here comes another one!" The contractions felt like waves of pressure—waves I had to ride. I would close my eyes and visualize a wall: up one side, on top of it, and then back to the ground. Ian stayed beside me and talked me through them.

At 4:30 p.m., after I had reached 3 centimeters dilation, I finally started active labor. I'd had approximately 17 hours of what they call "latent" or early labor. It sure felt real to me! I had been told that normally latent labor only lasts about six to eight hours. Lucky me.

I spent the next 11 hours dilating to the point where I could push. My membranes had not ruptured, although I could feel some amniotic fluid leaking out. I spent as much time as I could moving during those 11 hours. My apartment was configured in such a way that there was a circuit I could walk: through the living room, through the kitchen, through the hallway, and back into the living room. When I would have a contraction, I would hold onto the nearest person or piece of furniture, close my eyes, and try to let go of the pain, not fight it. The pain was amazing: my husband, who was still beside me, had to remind me to breathe for almost all of my contractions, because when they hit, I would instinctively clench my teeth and hold my breath, which made it worse. Breathing, deeply and regularly, *through* the pain was the best way to deal with it. I spent some time in the bathtub, where I found the pain less jarring, though no less intense.

MY HUSBAND HAD TO REMIND ME TO BREATHE, BECAUSE WHEN THE CONTRACTIONS HIT, I WOULD INSTINCTIVELY CLENCH MY TEETH AND HOLD MY BREATH, WHICH MADE IT WORSE.

I don't remember much about the transition phase, except that I had several contractions back to back and that Ian had to yell at me to breathe through them. I remember that Elizabeth checked my progress fairly often and that her examinations always caused the next contraction to be much more painful.

When I was 7 to 8 centimeters dilated, Elizabeth called Molly and asked her to come. She arrived at around 1:30 a.m. Soon after her arrival, I asked her to break my membranes, which she did while I was lying on my bedroom floor, surrounded by six friends. By this time, Eric, our baby's godfather, and our dear friends Jody and Lise were also there helping out. It was a real party.

The birth kit we had purchased from Molly had already been put to use. Someone prepared the bed by layering it with an old shower curtain, then receiving blankets, and then a set of old sheets on top. An oxygen tank stood in the corner, just in case. A birthing chair had been brought into the apartment and set up for me.

I was still on the floor, being cared for by all my friends. By this time, I was so tired. I know I could not have done it without them. One made sure I was getting enough liquids, another put cold cloths on my forehead, another put hot compresses on my belly (joy!), and the others held me while I contracted. Molly checked me after she broke my membranes and found that I had a small "lip" of cervix still in the way, which she moved. I don't remember feeling that. Then she left the room for a while and only returned when she could tell by my breathing that it was time for me to start pushing. Later, my husband told me that my sounds were gruntlike and huffy. I guess I was still unaware of my breathing.

I never experienced any overwhelming urge to push—I had to be told to do it. That amazes me. Anyway, I started pushing, in a semisitting position on the floor while still wearing my bathrobe. It was at this point that I think I no longer cared who saw what and I just relaxed as much as I could. I pushed in various positions: sitting on the toilet, sitting on the birthing chair, semisitting on my bed with my friend Jody holding me up from behind. (The birthing chair didn't work very well for me, because the baby wasn't moving down enough; so this position did nothing but cause my nether parts to swell considerably.)

They gave me oxygen and told me to push harder. By this time, I was exhausted. But the baby made her way down and crowned after an hour and a half of pushing. I realized then why the crowning stage is called the "ring of fire." It did sting, but that pales in comparison to the intensity of actually pushing. Pushing the baby out, I felt like I was using the same muscles as you do when you're having a bowel movement, though I remember feeling as if I was trying to push out my entire insides. I half expected to see my inner organs lying around me when it was all over.

I felt excited that I had gotten this far on my energy reserves. At the crowning, Molly invited me to touch the baby's head, which I did when my hand was placed between my legs. But mostly, I just wanted to get on with it.

When her head finally emerged, the baby made a 180-degree turn. This told Molly that the baby was stuck on my pubic

I HALF EXPECTED TO SEE MY INNER ORGANS LYING AROUND ME WHEN IT WAS ALL OVER.

bone, a situation called shoulder dystocia. So, after her head was completely out, Molly reached in and grabbed the baby's posterior shoulder and pulled her out. Ian caught her, amazed by how slippery she was.

In all, I had pushed for two hours, with my friend Christine snapping photographs all the way. Those two hours went by very quickly and felt more like 45 minutes.

When the baby was out on my belly, she was blue and her cord was not throbbing. I didn't know her sex. That seemed such a trivial fact, compared to the odyssey of the birth. But it clicked in my head suddenly and it occurred to me to ask. I was glad to hear it was a girl. Then I started to bleed quite a bit. I was so focused on the baby, my friends had to remind me to get back to my body's business—I still had a placenta to deliver. I don't remember much more after this point, except that they took the baby away and gave her oxygen. Less than five minutes later, my daughter was in my arms, and she was fine. I had stopped bleeding. And everyone cried with relief and joy. Then the neighbors, who didn't know I was having a baby in my apartment, banged on the wall (it was 5:30 a.m.!), giving us all a good laugh. Perhaps they thought we had been partying all night.

After the baby was born and my bleeding had stopped, I delivered the placenta with no problem. Molly offered to show it to me, but I said no thanks. She put it into a white plastic bag and stuck it in the freezer so that when it was disposed of, it wouldn't immediately attract the neighborhood wildlife! When I took it out of the freezer a week or so later, I was amazed at how heavy it was.

Rebekah Maya was 8 pounds, 7 ounces, and had a 14-inch head— and I had not torn! When she was breathing on her own, she was placed at my breast and began to nurse. I remember looking down at her and weeping, thinking, "Oh, my God, it's over! I have a baby!" I was overwhelmed, but euphoric. And yes, exhausted, like I'd just run up Mount Everest and down the other side!

After a while, Molly helped me into the bathroom, where she gave me a short but much-needed shower. I was trembling quite badly and had to hold onto the wall for support. Ian saw me in the shower when Molly was bathing me and said he was surprised that I still looked about six months pregnant. (I had been warned to expect that by my twin sister, who had given birth four months earlier.) When I got back into bed, there were clean sheets and fresh disposable pads waiting for me. The shot of Pitocin I had been given to stop the bleeding and start my uterus shrinking was working, so Molly was feeling okay about my recovery. Normally, she does not give the drug, as putting the baby to nurse right after birth will usually start the uterus shrinking. However, when there is excessive bleeding, Molly does what is necessary to stop it. She also gave me some herbal tea to drink.

WHEN I THANKED MY MIDWIFE FOR DELIVERING MY BABY, SHE CORRECTED ME, SAYING THAT *I* HAD DELIVERED MY BABY: SHE HAD JUST HELPED.

Then someone made a big breakfast for everyone. We ate our meal together and then everyone went home.

After 24 hours Molly came back to check on us and to teach us how to swaddle the baby, how to take care of her umbilicus, and to answer any questions we had. It was great to see Molly after it was all over—and yet all just beginning. When I thanked her for delivering my baby, she corrected me, saying that *I* had delivered my baby: she had just helped.

Giving birth at home was the most amazing thing I have ever done in my life. I did not use any drugs at all during the 25 hours of my labor. However, I do understand why some women would want them; there were a few contractions that I had to silently congratulate myself for getting through because I couldn't talk much. Apparently I grunted, moaned, and groaned, and perhaps spoke very fast, one- or two-word sentences. I know I kept telling myself that this was *productive* pain, that I'd have something miraculous at the end to show for it.

Ian was a great coach. He could tell when I was at the peak of a contraction and talk me through it. And even though he wasn't feeling well, and was becoming feverish himself during my long labor, he still managed to hold my hand and be enthusiastic for me and do whatever I needed whenever I needed it.

By the next morning though, he was quite ill with a viral infection. We were a fine pair! For the next few days, he slept on the couch, trying to get as much sleep as possible so he could be at my "beck and call." Some friends slept over to help out with the midnight changings and nursings. For a couple of days, I was so sore I had trouble moving easily. Other friends came by to cook for us, which I will remember with gratitude for as long as I live.

Having our friends there with us, sharing in the joy of welcoming our child into the world was the most beautiful aspect of it all. Their support and love made it possible for me to do it, even when, about 18 hours into it, I thought I just couldn't do it anymore. I think it was also because of them that it never occurred to me for one moment that anything could go wrong. They were good friends before, but since that day, we have been bonded for life.

A Big Sister Helps

Ashley was nine years old when she witnessed her sister's birth in a hospital in Fort Myers, Florida, where she lives and goes to school. When she's not playing with her sister, she likes to do all kinds of stuff with her friends.

I was at my friend's house, helping with their new baby because they needed a break sometimes, when my dad called on the phone. My friend said that she wasn't supposed to tell me but my mom's water had broken. (My dad didn't want her to tell me because he wanted to surprise me.)

So my dad came, and I got in the car, and we were driving down the road, and he said, "Mom's water broke." And I said, "I know." He said, "Oh, well, okay."

When we got home, Mom was in the bedroom, in bed. She had about four inches of towels under her and they were soaked through with water, so we took her to the hospital. She had had two false labors before this, so I didn't want to go this time since I was disappointed the other times and I kinda thought this might be another false labor. But the doctor said, "Get in here, right away," after her water broke, so I thought this might be it.

It was about 9:30 p.m. The front doors of the hospital were locked, so we had to go around to the emergency room entrance. They brought her a wheelchair and they pushed her to Labor and Delivery, to her room. The nurse checked her and said, "You're only 1 centimeter, but because your water broke, we have to admit you." Before the nurse left to find a room, I told her she was the nicest nurse ever for accepting my mom.

My mom had a really nice room in the hospital. It had a bed, a couch, and two chairs. My dad was on the couch, so I had to put the two chairs together and try to sleep on them. It was really hard. My legs were too long. I woke my mom and dad up when I tried to get comfortable because the chairs squeaked. My mom and dad told me I had to go to sleep, but, of course, I wanted to stay up and watch the monitors and everything. They had to listen to the baby's heart rate and watch Mom's contractions. But Mom and Dad said I had to go to sleep because it would be a long night, so we all slept.

But sometime in the night, Mom got sick. I woke up and saw she wasn't in her bed and I got scared, so I went into the bathroom to help her. I had to rip the monitors off her. I asked her, "Should I go get the nurse?" And she said, "Yeah." The nurse came in and walked into the bathroom, but Mom was already back in bed. My mom asked her, "Will you put the monitors back on me?" And she said, "Sure."

My dad told me later that he heard my mom moaning at about 1:00 a.m., and he got up and asked, "Are you okay?" and she said, "No." About 20 minutes later, I woke up. Mom was propped up in bed having a contraction. So I got up and got on her other side, and I held her hand.

At about 2:00 a.m., the nurse called the doctor. I kept wondering where he was, because he didn't come in. I thought he would be right there. But the nurse said Mom had to build up her contractions before the doctor would come. By then, she was dilated about 5 centimeters.

I was still standing there, holding her hand. She was having a lot of contractions and they came really fast. I was a little bit worried because she was in so much pain from how hard the contractions were hitting her. After about 45 minutes, the doctor came in. They brought out this really big cart with all the little scissors and stuff, and I was looking at that thinking "*Ouch*" 'cause I knew it all had something to do with her. Then the doctor went back out and that made me even madder. I just thought he should be there because what if she right away went into the pushing stage?

By then she was about 6 or 7 centimeters, and this went on for what seemed like a really long time, but it was probably only about 20 minutes, before she climbed another centimeter or two. The doctor came back in and checked her, and she was 9 centimeters. He said, "Well, you have to reach 10."

My dad didn't want to leave my mom, so I kept having to go out and tell the nurse, "She wants to push! She wants to push!" And the nurse would say, "Well, tell her she can't." And I would say, "No, don't tell me that."

About 15 minutes later, the doctor came back in and said, "Okay, you're ready to push. Now, on every contraction, push as hard as you can and as long as you can."

I was still standing there beside her, and she was holding one of my hands, and my fingers were turning purple. She said the contractions were back to back. She pushed for two hours, holding my hand. Sometimes she got really hot and asked the nurse to take off the monitors and her nightgown. After all, they *knew* she was having contractions, so they didn't need that monitor. When the doctor came back into the room, he was surprised to see her naked. But he didn't say anything.

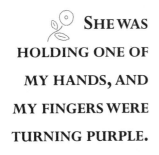 **SHE WAS HOLDING ONE OF MY HANDS, AND MY FINGERS WERE TURNING PURPLE.**

It was hard to get my sister's head out so they wanted to use this vacuum, but it was broken. So the staff scattered all over the hospital looking for a missing part. They couldn't find the part, so the nurse came back in and said, "Sorry, we can't find it." They decided to put the suction cup on her head anyway just to hold her so she wouldn't slip back in, because she had been coming out and going back in the whole time. The doctor had to just hold the suction cup by hand.

They set up the squatting bars on the bed and my mom squatted on the bed. They got her head out with my mom pushing. My mom put her own head under the bar so she could see, and I was standing right there, almost where the doctor was, so I saw too. The baby's head came out, and she turned it to the side and blood went in her ear and her nose. That was the scariest part because it was blood. Yuck! And she had vernix, too. A few more pushes, maybe five more, and she came out: Anna.

It was kinda strange because it wasn't like I thought it would be.

Both my mom and the doctor were wrong about what they thought would happen. The doctor had said that usually the second one is easier, and this wasn't. And my mom had said there wasn't much blood when I was born, and there was a ton of blood with Anna.

My mom lay down on the bed with my sister on her tummy, and the doctor cut the cord. Then I went with the nurse to weigh Anna and get her measured, and the nurse did something to Anna's foot to make her scream. I think she weighed 6 pounds 11 ounces. She was 18 inches long. She was born at 4:28 a.m.

The nurse put her under the lamps and wrapped her up. She gave Anna back to my mom to try to nurse, but my mom couldn't get Anna close enough because of the blankets she was wrapped in, so they took them off. Anna kept trying to get her arms out anyway.

I was excited the whole time, right from the moment when we got to the hospital. I'd been there before, to visit babies who were brothers and sisters of my friends, but I'd never brought a baby home before. When Anna came out, it was—well, the whole thing was definitely a once-in-a-lifetime experience.

A Hospital Birth (1959)

*Wenda Fay is the younger sister of Pam
(Lucas's mom, whose birth story is told on pages 78–88).
Pam and Wenda Fay's mother, who died in 1976,
left behind this account of her fourth, and youngest, child's birth
in a Philadelphia hospital in 1959. "As I read through the story
of Wenda's birth," Pam writes, "an emotion approaching pity
overwhelms me as I compare my own birthing experience,
where I was in control, to that of my mother, where the doctor and
hospital staff made all the decisions, even down to when
she would be able to see and touch her newborn baby."*

I was hoping very much that this baby would decide to arrive on March 15, my birthday. During the last month or six weeks I was uncomfortable many times with false labor pains and was beginning to feel quite uneasy as each time I wondered if they were going to develop into true labor. We painted the living room over that weekend and Mum and I worked very hard cleaning it up and putting it all back in order. I shampooed the rug while Mum and Gordon [her husband] did the furniture-moving.

I saw Dr. N. at 4:00 p.m. on March 17 for my regular appointment. He made an internal examination and said I was all ready for labor. He suggested that I take castor oil between 9:00 and 10:00 that evening and labor would surely follow very soon afterward. At first I thought he was kidding, but that was his prescription in all seriousness. So I made one more trip to the grocery store on the way home and stocked up as well as I could for the family while I would be away, and bought the castor oil. I spent that evening drawing designs for the birth announcement, finishing some mending, and so on.

At 9:20 p.m. I took the castor oil and followed it with a drink of orange juice. By 9:40, I was making trips to the bathroom and was mighty uncomfortable. By 10:15, my intestinal tract was finally emptied and I stopped making trips to the bathroom. I was very tired by then. At 10:30 p.m., the contractions started but they were very weak and scarcely noticeable. I left the light on to try to keep myself awake to time them. They were so mild that they scarcely roused me but they were coming every five minutes or less. Dr. N.'s instructions were to call him as soon as they were of increasing severity. I had asked him that afternoon how long a labor he thought I might have and he was completely noncommittal, indicating it would probably be about average.

By midnight, they were still mild cramps, just as in the beginning, but I decided that before it got any later I wanted to get Dr. N.'s advice, especially since I had taken the castor oil he had prescribed. I talked to his answering service at 12:05 a.m. and told them I was having mild cramps every five minutes but that they were so mild they weren't even making me squirm. A few minutes later the nurse at the hospital called me back and said the doctor wanted me to come into the hospital.

Halfway to the hospital, the cramps stopped entirely. I told Gordon I thought they would be sending me home again. Then a little before we arrived real labor started.

I was having about the fourth good contraction as we reached the hospital. I knew I would be staying. Just as we walked in the door of the lobby my water broke with a deluge. I sat myself down in the wheelchair as soon as I could get to it. I think if I hadn't, this baby might have been born in the lobby.

I reached the preparation room at 1:00 a.m. and tried to undress. I got my skirt and blouse off, pushed my straps down, crawled onto the bed, and the nurse came to the rescue. We didn't even have all of my clothes off before Dr. N. was checking me. He took just one glance and said, "Look what we have here! Get the traveling gas mask and call the anesthetist." We were still getting my shoes and socks off when the cart arrived to take me to the delivery room.

A nurse tried to shave me on the delivery table and asked me not to push. I assured her I wasn't. Then she stopped shaving suddenly and said, "That's all I can do." The anesthetist arrived and put a different type mask onto my face. I closed my eyes part of the time to get the full benefit of the gas but I could hear what was going on and I could feel a good bit, too. I felt a wonderful relief from the terrific pressure when the baby was pushed out, and then I heard her cry. They told me later that she arrived at 1:07 a.m., seven minutes after I got to the preparation room. I felt the afterbirth plop out. And then I was told to hold still while the doctor stitched me—internal stitches only. They told me it was a girl before I was able to see the clock. It was 1:20 when I could see the clock and I

could also see the baby's arm and knee in a basket near me. I asked to see her and the nurse brought her over just as soon as she was finished with the job she was doing. I held her across my stomach. She was naked except for a wee square of blanket around her back. I asked the nurse if she was warm enough and she said, "Yes."

I asked to see the afterbirth but it was already disposed of. They took the baby away when they said the doctor was ready to take her out to show Gordon. They said he was completely dumbfounded that the baby was here already. Finally they finished squeezing my uterus and pushing blood clots out to their satisfaction and I was taken to my room. We stopped by the solarium on the way and talked to

I COULD ALSO SEE THE BABY'S ARM AND KNEE IN A BASKET NEAR ME. I ASKED TO SEE HER AND THE NURSE BROUGHT HER OVER JUST AS SOON AS SHE WAS FINISHED WITH THE JOB SHE WAS DOING.

Gordon. After I was in bed, he came in and we talked for quite a while.

It was 3:00 a.m. when Gordon reached home again. Mum asked him how long the doctor thought it would be until the baby was born!

They gave me a sleeping pill but I didn't sleep well. However, I sort of caught up with my sleep by taking numerous naps during that day and the next. The second day I awakened feeling nauseated. I thought it was from being so hungry. We were awakened at 5:15 a.m. and breakfast didn't come until 8:00. This morning I also felt weak and shaky. I ate breakfast even though I didn't feel quite right. Of course, I lost it again about an hour later. Dr. N.'s substitute looked at me that morning and suggested I eat lightly at noon. I did, even though my appetite was pretty good. Supper came at 5:00 and tasted horrible—who would want broiled halibut and spinach after a queasy day? (That's what I'd ordered the previous day so I can't blame the hospital.) I realized that my eyes were burning before they brought out the babies again so I asked the nurse to take my temperature. She didn't tell me why, but she promptly called Dr. N. and I was told he'd be there in an hour. I called Gord and told him I was sick. I asked him to be here when the doctor came and to bring me some saltines.

Dr. N. concluded that I didn't tolerate codeine and that I was nauseated from the pills they'd given me for the afterbirth cramps. He thought the fever must be from my milk coming in, as he could find no other cause for it. However, he did have me take sulfa tablets or some such thing for the remainder of my stay in the hospital. I was catheterized that evening, too, so they could take a urinalysis.

Friday I felt so weak that any bit of exertion or walking around made me burst into tears. I felt much better by Saturday, and I was glad for the extra rest. Saturday night my milk came in so suddenly I was engorged to the point where I was miserable in any position and couldn't sleep. The next morning, Sunday, the fourth day, I was discharged, the same as all the other maternity patients.

It's All in Your Head

Cheryll was a 32-year-old executive secretary when her first
child was born, in a hospital in Scottsdale, Arizona. Her
husband, a finance manager, was 37. Cheryll used a
form of self-hypnosis during labor and feels that more
women should know about this option.

A few weeks before my due date, I received a call from an older cousin who had given birth to her second child within the past year. She was the first and only person who spoke to me about preparing for a positive, natural birthing experience. My cousin told me of her experience with a midwife, and I listened with enthusiasm. She was the only person I spoke to who didn't tell me to "go with the epidural" so I could enjoy childbirth.

I had been concerned about the epidural all along. I had had difficulty getting pregnant, and the baby was so precious to me, I did not want to take any chances with its health. I worried that the drug wouldn't be good for the baby. In my seventh month, I had read about epidurals and painkillers in *What to Expect When You're Expecting* and the basic advice was to try to avoid drugs if possible. I also wasn't convinced I could push the baby out if I was numb from the waist down. I had heard of many women who had done this, but I had also heard of some who couldn't. I really wanted to avoid having a suction or forceps delivery if I could.

So when my doctor suggested I use the epidural, since it was my first time, I told him I really wanted to try without it and see how it felt. He was supportive of my decision. After that, I went around half-jokingly telling everyone that I wanted a four-hour labor with no epidural. It turns out, that's basically what I had. Today, I wonder if it happened that way because I focused on that thought so much before the actual birth. Since the birth, I've become a believer in the power of our minds.

To prepare for delivery, I exercised and ate a nutritious diet. In my eighth month, I began to look around for books on meditative techniques that would help me to work with the labor instead of against it, to help me open myself to an instinctive knowledge of labor and birth. The first book I read made so much sense to me, it became the only one I used: *Mind Over Labor* by Carl Jones. This author advocated using imagery to help your body birth. One of the suggested images was that of a flower opening. When I read it, I thought of the time-lapse photography I'd seen of a beautiful white rose blooming. I came to believe that my body knew what to do. But I had made no firm decision about exactly what imagery I would use when the time came.

My first contractions woke me up at 3:30 a.m. Easter morning. They were very regular, about 8 or 10 minutes apart, and I felt them down low on my uterus, like menstrual cramps. They were very manageable, but I was so excited, I didn't go back to sleep. Since it was only one week before my due date, I was pretty sure this was real labor.

I didn't know what to expect. Because I thought I might be rushing to the hospital at some point, I eventually got up and took a shower, put on my makeup, and made myself presentable. When my husband awoke, my contractions hadn't changed, but they hadn't stopped, either. So we got on with our day.

We went out to breakfast, took a two-hour walk, then had some lunch. At lunch, a hard contraction came that made me stop eating. My husband said, "Are you okay?" And I replied, "Well, that one made my eyes water. It was that hard." But they weren't all like that. We had my bag packed and in the trunk of the car, so we knew we were ready to go to the hospital the minute we wanted to. At that point, I still felt like everything was manageable, so we went to the movies, as planned, and then returned home. We spent the afternoon preparing Easter dinner (all the while timing my contractions).

As the contractions became stronger, I remember having to stop what I was doing in the kitchen, grab onto the counter and bend over a little, close my eyes, do some Lamaze breathing, and wait for the contraction to pass. I could now feel a real tightening and hardening of my uterus. The contractions were lasting a minute at least and were gradually coming closer together. By 6:00 p.m., they were five minutes apart. That was my official signal to call the doctor.

We arrived at the hospital sometime after 7:00 p.m. Since it was Easter, there was no anesthesiologist on the premises, and they asked me if they should call one in, as it would take some time to make the arrangements. At this point, I said, "No, thank you."

Once I was in the Labor and Delivery room and hooked up to the external monitor, I reclined in an easy chair and, during a contraction, heard the nurse tell my husband that she had never seen anyone in labor so calm. I stayed in that chair for about four hours, lost in the power of my mind and body. I expected my body to know what to do instinctively, the way a baby knows how to suck, and I thought succumbing to labor would be much better than fighting or fearing it. I got lost in my imagery, and together with the breathing I'd learned in the Lamaze classes, that's how I dealt with the pain. During the Lamaze classes, I did not feel at all comfortable with the breathing I was being taught. But in the middle of my labor, I found myself using it, and it worked perfectly for me.

> **DURING THE LAMAZE CLASSES, I DID NOT FEEL AT ALL COMFORTABLE WITH THE BREATHING I WAS BEING TAUGHT. BUT IN THE MIDDLE OF MY LABOR, I FOUND MYSELF USING IT, AND IT WORKED PERFECTLY FOR ME.**

I don't know if you can really plan which imagery to use. I didn't. For me, the image of the opening flower bud popped into my head right at the beginning of the heavy contractions, and it felt right so I used it the whole time. But this was not something I "saw" or visualized. I actually felt that I *became* the flower. I was trying to feel my pelvis and vagina opening like a flower to let the baby out. This helped me to accept the pain. I also had my husband watch the monitor and tell me with each contraction when it had peaked. I used that information to help me coordinate my breathing efforts, and I focused very much on the rhythm of my breathing. This helped me to not panic. The contractions were lasting much longer than I had realized they would.

I wore the monitor the entire time I was in the chair, so the nurse, the doctor (who had arrived within 30 minutes of my arrival and stayed with me the entire time), and my husband could see when I was near transition. Since my water hadn't yet broken, the doctor decided to break it himself while I was still in the chair. This was a bit of a juggle, but I was so comfortable in the chair, I really didn't want to get out of it. As soon as the water broke, the contractions became much stronger and lasted much longer. During one of these contractions, I shook my head back and forth because it seemed like the contraction wouldn't stop. The duration of these contractions surprised me. I became a bit scared, and thought briefly about the epidural. At that point, I turned to my doctor and asked, "Do you think I can do it?" He said, "Oh, yes. You can do this." That was all I needed to hear.

When I felt the urge to push, I had to move to the bed. The bed had a bottom that dropped away and a head that was elevated. I put my legs over these stirruplike poles on the sides of the bed and grabbed the handles on each side of me to hold onto while pushing. (My arms were quite sore the next day.)

The urge to push was overwhelming. I couldn't not do it. Before each push, I would take two cleansing breaths. Because I was pushing the baby out much faster than the doctor thought prudent, he gave me an episiotomy. I don't know exactly how long I pushed, but I'm sure I wasn't on the bed for more than half an hour.

I am proud to say I can remember the feeling of my daughter's head passing through me, as well as the remainder of her 9-pound, 13-ounce body. During the last part of the birth, I was elevated to a state where my focus was intent on one thing: bringing my baby safely into the world. The doctor asked me if I wanted a mirror to watch, and I had to break my concentration to answer, "No." I felt I couldn't leave my task. In retrospect, I was so focused the entire time I was in labor, I was just doing, not thinking. The voices of encouragement from my husband, the doctor, and the nurse seemed to come from somewhere far away. I lost all care or thought for anything but my ultimate goal.

I WAS SO FOCUSED THE ENTIRE TIME I WAS IN LABOR, I WAS JUST DOING, NOT THINKING.

The only disappointing thing was that as soon as my daughter was born, they immediately took her away to another table, cleaned and measured her, and brought her back to me all swaddled. I missed holding her naked. When I did hold her, I noticed how large she was and asked immediately how much she weighed. I am six feet tall, so I guess it shouldn't have been too surprising that she was such a big girl. And no doubt my size helped me to birth such a large baby.

I truly believe that I could have never pushed out that baby had it not been for the fact that I could feel the urge to push and was able to succumb to my body's instinct. Amazingly, I was very calm throughout the labor. I really had no time to be screaming at the nurse or yelling at my husband. I think keeping sight of my goal made everything else just fall away. I wasn't ever scared. I went into labor very informed and confident. Of course, I knew something could go wrong, but because I felt so secure with my doctor and the hospital, the thought never entered my head during the labor. I kept a positive attitude the entire time.

You need to be true to yourself, ask lots of questions, and make your own choices. I think women need to know that you can handle the task your body and nature present you with.

Glossary

anterior position The birth position in which the baby enters the pelvis facing the mother's spine, with its back against her uterine wall and its face to the rear. The most common and easiest position for birth.

antibiotic ointment Applied to newborn's eyes; required treatment within two hours of birth in most states. The purpose is to guard against eye infections that can lead to blindness. The most common of these infections is gonorrhea, which often is symptomless and not always detected by tests.

APGAR rating Developed by Dr. Virginia Apgar, an anesthesiologist, to judge how well a baby is functioning at birth and how well and how quickly it adapts to its new environment. The test is given twice, at one minute after birth and again at five minutes after birth. The test rates the same five things both times: heart rate, respiratory effort, muscle tone, reflex irritability, and skin color as an indication of circulation (in non-Caucasian babies, the color of the whites of the eyes, the mucous membranes of the mouth, the lips, palms, hands, and soles of the feet are examined).

back labor Labor in which the baby is facing forward instead of backward, and its spine presses against the mother's spine with each contraction, creating extreme pain in the mother's lower back.

BBP The baseline blood pressure reading determined during pregnancy to be the mother's "normal" pressure, used during labor to evaluate her laboring condition. A diastolic increase of 20 points or more during labor might indicate a problem. (*see* blood pressure)

bilirubin The baby has more red blood cells in utero than it needs after birth. During the first week of life, the baby must break down these excess red blood cells and excrete them through the urine, feces, skin, and lungs. One of the products of this breakdown is bilirubin, an orange or yellow substance in the bile. The baby's liver picks up this unnecessary substance and converts it to a non-toxic form that is easily excreted. (*see* jaundice)

birthing bed A hospital bed that can be adjusted to aid a woman during delivery. The bottom of the bed can be removed, the head of the bed can be raised, stirrups may be attached to the sides, and it is high enough to facilitate a caregiver's view. Squat bars can be attached on some models. (*see* squat bars)

birthing center Two kinds operate in the United States. A hospital-affiliated center may be located within a hospital or adjacent to it and is staffed by midwives who work with the obstetrics unit of the hospital or with an obstetrics group in the area and have privileges at the hospital. The midwives provide all prenatal care, and they deliver all uncomplicated vaginal births. These centers often provide more pain relief alternatives to laboring women than hospitals do, such as tubs or Jacuzzis or large air-filled balls to rock on during contractions. The birthing rooms are usually like hospital rooms, with adjustable steel-frame birthing beds and linoleum floors, but they may also have private bathrooms and an extra bed for your partner to sleep on.

A free-standing birthing center is not necessarily affiliated with an obstetrics practice or with a hospital. It is more homelike and often is located in a former home. The center is run by midwives, and some are owned by midwives. Depending on state requirements, midwives either informally consult with or are legally associated with a local obstetrician to whom they can refer prenatal patients when necessary and call for backup dur-

ing labor if complications develop. The birthing rooms usually look like bedrooms, have private baths, and have a kitchen nearby. Often they contain Jacuzzis, birthing pools, and other non-traditional labor aids and birth options.

blood pressure The force exerted by the blood against the arterial walls. Systolic pressure (the first number) is the pumping measurement, taken when the heart is at its maximum contraction. The diastolic pressure (the second number) is the resting measurement, i.e., the measurement taken when the heart is relaxed between beats. An increase of 20 points or more in the diastolic pressure reading might indicate problems in a pregnancy.

bloody show Also called pink show. During pregnancy, the cervix is closed by a gelatinous plug of mucus. As labor nears and the cervix begins to efface and dilate, the plug begins to dislodge. As it does, a woman may notice a mucous discharge tinged with pink or brown blood. The show can be more blood than mucus, or vice versa, and is an indication that the body is getting ready for labor, though it may still be a few weeks away.

Braxton Hicks contractions Mild, irregular, pre-labor uterine contractions that can begin as early as the seventh month in first-time pregnancies and even earlier in subsequent pregnancies. The contraction begins at the top of the uterus and spreads downward. Some women can feel them as they occur; others feel them only if they place their hand on their uterus as it becomes hard and then relaxes. These contractions exercise the uterus, bringing blood to it and preparing it for labor. Some doctors believe that Braxton Hicks contractions help efface and dilate the cervix.

breech position When the baby is presenting itself for birth in other than a head down position. This occurs in only 3 percent of pregnancies. Complete breech is the baby sitting cross-legged at the bottom of the uterus, with his buttocks presenting first. If the baby is frank breech, her legs are straight up, with her feet near her face and her buttocks presenting first. Footling breech (very rare) occurs when the baby's foot or feet present first; and knee breech (even more rare) occurs when the baby's knee presents first.

colostrum The yellow or creamy liquid that precedes breast milk. It can leak from breasts before birth. A baby is not born hungry, and colostrum is not intended to supply nutrition. Rather, it prepares and stimulates the baby's digestive tract to do its work. It is high in vitamins A and E, contains antibodies, and has twice the protein of mature breast milk. If the baby nurses at birth and during the days before the milk comes in, the colostrum does two things: it breaks down the mucus in the baby's digestive tract, preparing the passageways for milk, and it clears the meconium from the bowels. Flushing the bowels of meconium also clears the tract of bilirubin that is contained in the meconium. A baby who reabsorbs too much bilirubin develops jaundice. (*see* jaundice)

crowning The point during birth when the top of the baby's head becomes visible at the lips of the vagina.

dilation The action of opening the cervix for birth. The size of the opening is measured in centimeters from 0 to 10, with 10 indicating complete dilation.

doula A professional labor assistant, hired to care for and monitor a laboring woman. Many couples find the doula's training reassuring. A trained doula makes certain that the woman does not become dehydrated, that she eats as much as she needs, that she is supported emotionally, and that she is physically as comfortable as possible. She is able to judge the quality and progress of labor, often working with and reporting to a midwife. Some doulas stay for the birth and/or return after the birth to assist the new mother and father.

dropping *See* lightening

edema Swelling. Swelling is normal during pregnancy, and most women have some swelling. The pregnant body produces extra blood for the fetus and placenta, and extra fluid is retained to protect the woman from going into shock during birth and its subsequent bloodloss. However, anything more than mild edema should be reported to a caregiver. Severe edema can be an indication of kidney problems or other complications.

effacement During pregnancy, the cervix closes, wrinkling into itself and bunching to form a very narrow, short canal into the uterus. Shortly before labor starts, this canal or neck begins to soften and to flatten out, so that the cervix is again a round, soft shape. This process is measured by caregivers in percentages, from 0 to 100, with 100 being full effacement.

epidural A type of local anesthestic that numbs the nerves that carry pain messages from the lower part of the body to the brain. Using a small, thin catheter taped to the woman's back, the anesthetic is injected in the epidural space (the area just outside the membrane that covers the spinal fluid) between two vertebrae near the base of the spinal column. Epidurals are usually given after 6 centimeters dilation, though some doctors administer them earlier. If it is started too early, an epidural can slow down labor. Because it can cause a drop in maternal blood pressure, which reduces the amount of oxygen that the fetus receives, the process must include fetal monitoring and, for the mother, gauging blood pressure every 15 to 30 minutes and administering an IV hydrating solution.

episiotomy An incision made in the perineum muscle to enlarge the vaginal opening. It is made in one of two ways—either straight down from the vagina toward the anus, called a median, or downward but at an angle away from the vagina, called a medio-lateral. Many American doctors perform episiotomies routinely in order to avoid tearing of the perineum, but there are alternative ways to stretch the perineum, including massage and warm compresses.

false labor Also known as prodromal labor, occurs when the mother has the symptoms of labor without any noticeable changes in the cervix. Contractions may be irregular, they may subside if the mother walks around, and their intensity may diminish as time passes. False labor is probably a kind of warm-up exercise for the body—it may help soften the cervix—and should not be dismissed as useless. The main difference between actual labor and prodromal labor is that once labor begins in earnest, it usually does not stop and it does intensify over time.

fetal monitor An instrument that measures uterine contractions and fetal heart rate during labor. The monitor may be external, in the form of a belt fastened around the mother's abdomen, or internal, in the form of an electrode attached to the baby's scalp.

fontanels Also known as soft spots; the membranous spaces in an infant's skull, where the bones have not yet fused. The largest fontanel, located at the top of the head, is also called the baby's "soft spot." Another fontanel is located at the rear of the head. Because the infant's skull is not completely ossified at birth, it is able to compress slightly on its way down the birth canal. This compression often results in a cone-shape skull at birth.

forceps delivery Forceps are large, curved tongs. The two sides of the tongs are put into the vagina separately and slipped around each side of the baby's head. The tongs are locked into their opened position by the doctor, who pulls the baby out by the head.

frank breech position *See* breech position

gestational diabetes A temporary condition precipitated by hormonal changes in which the mother's body does not produce enough insulin to handle the increased blood sugar levels of pregnancy. Symptoms include excessive amounts of sugar in the mother's urine, unusual thirst, frequent urination, and fatigue. Uncontrolled diabetes results in too much sugar in the mother's blood, which will then enter the placenta and affect the fetus. This is a serious condition that must be treated by a physician.

induction of labor Labor medically brought on by administering Pitocin (*see* oxytocin) to the mother via an intravenous drip. Induction can occur for several reasons: to reduce risk of infection after the rupture of membranes, to deliver a baby who is overdue, or to ensure the health of both mother and child when conditions of diabetes, hypertension, or toxemia are present.

jaundice Yellow discoloration of the skin and eyes. In a newborn, jaundice is the result of an excess of bilirubin, an orange or yellow substance (*see* bilirubin). A baby is born with an excess of red blood cells. During the first week of life, the baby must break them down in order to excrete them. Bilirubin is a byproduct of this breakdown of red blood cells. When the baby's liver cannot catch up with converting the bilirubin to a nontoxic, excretable substance, a high level remains and jaundice occurs. Treatment of jaundice can be performed at home or in the hospital and includes phototherapy (periodically placing the baby under lights or in sunshine) and providing extra fluids, but treatment must occur under a pediatrician's care. Usually jaundice is harmless, but untreated, high levels of the unconverted bilirubin can damage the baby's nervous system and brain cells.

latching on Connecting the baby's mouth, tongue, and lips to the breast for feeding. Baby must be sucking on part of areola as well as the nipple in order to compress the milk glands and to avoid causing sore nipples. Her lips should surround the area, and her tongue should be beneath the breast, pulling the breast toward her with each suck.

latent labor The first stage of labor, during which the cervix becomes completely effaced and dilates to 3 centimeters.

lightening Also called dropping or engagement; occurs when the baby's presenting part, usually its head, settles into the pelvis. This occurs two or three weeks before labor in first pregnancies, and may not occur until early in labor in subsequent pregnancies. The caregiver will confirm the baby's position. After lightening, the woman may notice it is easier to breathe, and/or the woman may feel increased pressure on her pubic bone and a need to urinate more frequently due to the increased pressure on her blad-

der. The progress of the baby's descent into the pelvis is measured by centimeters and the positions are called stations. (*see* station)

meconium A greenish-brown substance in the fetal intestine that is passed soon after birth as the baby's first stool. Though not common, sometimes the baby passes meconium while still in-utero, especially if he or she is overdue. This stains the amniotic fluid, which is usually pale and clear, and may indicate a distressed baby. If the baby inhales or swallows any meconium prior to or during birth, a serious infection may result. Any signs of meconium staining in the amniotic fluid should be reported to your caregiver.

midwife A person trained to assist women in uncomplicated vaginal delivery. Three types of midwives practice in this country: certified nurse midwives (CNMs) who have completed both medical training as a registered nurse and certified training in midwifery; certified midwives (CMs) who have been trained at a midwifery school and received certification in midwifery; and lay midwives who have not completed certified training but who have served an apprenticeship.

A midwife's approach may differ from a doctor's in several ways. First, the midwife generally has more time to spend with each patient and strives to develop a personal relationship in order to better understand the mother's needs later, during birth. A midwife's training emphasizes allowing the woman to make decisions during her labor, and as long as everything is proceeding well, the midwife will accommodate the mother's wishes during labor. She will also stay with a patient for much of the labor as well as the delivery. Midwives are committed to nonintervention although they (especially the C.N.M.s) are thoroughly trained in medical technology. Certified nurse midwives can administer some pain relief (though not epidurals, which must be administered by an anesthesiologist). Generally, midwives are more flexible about procedures and positions during labor. Many of their techniques are not taught to doctors in medical school, so a midwife can present a pregnant and laboring woman with more choices in her care and delivery. Midwives cannot perform cesarean sections.

mucous plug A gelatinous plug of mucus that seals the cervical opening during pregnancy, both protecting it from external contamination and preventing the loss of amniotic fluid. The loss of this plug is one of the first signs of the onset of labor. A woman may discover a chunk of blood-stained mucus in her underpants or the toilet, or she may never see it at all. This can occur a week or more before contractions begin. (*see* bloody show)

non-stress test (NST) An in utero assessment of the baby's responsiveness and movement. This test is usually administered when the baby is overdue or when the caregiver suspects the baby is distressed. The woman sits or lies down with a fetal monitor belt around her waist and indicates each time she feels the baby move. The monitor measures the fetal heart rate along with any uterine activity, displaying the measurements on both a screen and a printout.

oxytocin A pituitary hormone secreted during childbirth to stimulate contractions and milk production. Synthetic oxytocics are used to induce labor or to speed up a slow labor. Pitocin is the most commonly used oxytocic.

perineum The area of skin and muscle between the vulva and the anus. This muscle must stretch during birth to allow the baby's head to emerge.

Pitocin A synthetic oxytocic used to induce or speed up labor. (*see* oxytocin)

posterior birth position When the baby's head enters the pelvis with the back of the skull pointing toward the mother's back, pressing its head into the mother's lower back. This position can be more painful to the mother than the anterior birth position and can lessen the urge to push because the baby's head is not as well applied to the cervix.

preeclampsia Also called toxemia, this is a complication of pregnancy that occurs in 5 to 10 percent of pregnancies, often between weeks 20 and 24. It is initially characterized by high blood pressure, edema, and high levels of protein in the urine. This is a serious condition that can compromise the baby's and the mother's health. Medical treatment is necessary to control the symptoms, especially the high blood pressure. When the blood is rushing too quickly through the arteries, the placenta cannot absorb sufficient nutrients and the baby will not develop to its full potential.

preterm labor Premature labor, which begins between weeks 20 and 37.

prodromal labor *See* false labor

pudendal block An anesthetic injected into the pudendal nerve in the vagina or buttocks. This numbs the vagina and perineum and is often used with a forceps delivery. While it dulls the urge to push, the mother can still feel the baby move down the birth canal and can push when told to.

ring of fire A stinging, burning sensation produced by the baby's stretching the outlet of the birth canal. This can be felt just before or during crowning. (*see* crowning)

spinal block An anesthetic injected in the same manner as an epidural, but instead of being placed in the epidural space surrounding the spinal cord, it is injected directly into the spinal fluid. This method delivers the anesthetic immediately and within seconds results in both numbness and paralysis up to the waist. A spinal block is often used in cesarean sections because of its rapid and thorough effect. The mother must lie flat for four to eight hours after delivery to avoid getting a spinal headache.

squat bars Also known as roll bars or pushing bars, they are attached to the side or end of a bed. Facing the bars and holding onto them, a woman in the pushing stage can roll forward onto her knees to lean and push during a contraction. Squat bars are designed with a low step that the mother uses as a seat so she can sit back and rest between pushes.

stages of childbirth The three stages of childbirth are labor, delivery of the baby, and delivery of the placenta.

stages of labor Labor is divided into several stages. The first is pre-labor. The baby's presenting part may settle into the mother's pelvis, and the mother may experience Braxton Hicks contractions, notice an increase in vaginal mucus, experience a spurt of energy known as the nesting instinct, and/or feel premenstrual symptoms. She may also experience a period of false labor when she has contractions. None of these changes in her body will result in dilation of her cervix; they are all preparations for labor. The next phase is early first-stage labor, when productive contractions begin. The contractions increase in duration and frequency and result in dilation of the cervix, usually to 3 centimeters. This is followed by active, or late first-stage, labor, with productive contractions that bring the woman to 7 centimeters' dilation. First-stage labor ends with transition, the most difficult part, when the cervical dilation increases from 7 centimeters to 10 centimeters, complete dilation. Second-stage labor occurs when the mother pushes the baby down the birth canal and out. Third-stage labor is when the mother expels the placenta.

station One of eight numbers used to describe the degree to which the baby has descended into the mother's pelvis. The stations range from -4, indicating that descent has not begun, to +4, indicating that descent is complete and the baby's presenting part (usually its head) is fully engaged in the mother's pelvis.

suctioning Performed by a caregiver with a tiny sucking device immediately upon an infant's birth to remove any fluids (amniotic, meconium, vernix) from her mouth or nasal passages. Clearing the the baby's airways enables the baby to take her first few breaths fully and eliminates the possibility of choking. Not all babies need to be suctioned.

transition The third and last stage of labor. *See* stages of labor

transverse position The position in which the baby is lying horizontally across the mother's uterus. This position does not present a problem during pregnancy. During labor, however, it warrants a cesarean section.

vernix A fatty white substance secreted by oil glands in the skin of the fetus; it covers the skin and protects it from becoming waterlogged during the last few months of soaking in amniotic fluid. Eventually the vernix dissolves; this is why early or on-time babies have more vernix than late babies and why late babies tend to be more wrinkled.

vitamin K A fat-soluble vitamin essential for the formation of prothrombin, a substance necessary for the clotting of blood. Some hospitals give the baby vitamin K either right after birth or within a few days of it.

These pages are reserved for the most important story of all:
Yours

L · A · B · O · R   D · A · Y